Dr. Chrisanne Gordon, M~~~~ ~~~ ~~~~~~ ~~~~~

Foreword by Scott C. Livingston, PhD

TURN THE LIGHTS ON!

A PHYSICIAN'S PERSONAL JOURNEY

from the Darkness of Traumatic Brain Injury (TBI)
to Hope, Healing, and Recovery

PRAISE FOR *TURN THE LIGHTS ON!*

"I truly believe Dr. Gordon has cracked the code on TBI. This book is going to save millions of lives including veterans and former athletes. Turn the Lights On! is a must read for anyone who loves veterans and athletes like I do."

Jonathan Wells, J. Wells Media Group

"The personal approach in which Dr. Chrisanne Gordon writes is so powerful that it immediately draws you into a seemingly paradoxical world of amazing terror and hope. The brain, we learn, heals in chunks, not gradually. We learn that traumatic brain injury is not a mind hurt, but a brain hurt. Medication and surgery aren't the answer, but tenacious patience and committed compassion are. As both a victim and observer of TBI, Dr. Gordon communicates the importance of healing not just the injury, but the whole person. Ideally, the salvation of those who suffer from TBI including veterans, athletes, and others, will come when all stakeholders in the health care continuum come together and join forces in the fight, God willing."

Montgomery J. Granger, Major, US Army, Retired

"As a combat veteran, I can attest that Dr. Chrisanne Gordon is an ardent advocate who also has experienced her own TBI. This book illuminates the subject and conveys the journey that had led Dr. Gordon to pivot towards a new direction. She has the propensity of being a leader, and as such addresses the obstacles—both legislative and medical—to achieve a successful mission—to educate, properly diagnose, and treat TBI."

Wendell Guillermo
Software Developer and OIF Combat Veteran

"In her fabulous book, Chrisanne Gordon, MD, shows off her genius through her innate ability to look into her own brain-injured mind and recount her thoughts and emotions as she goes through the emotions and thoughts from the moment of brain injury to the moments of re-discovery of 'herself' as she used to be. She is a physician who has discovered one of the innermost secrets of caring for the patients–the physician must assume and carry some of the burden of pain, injury, and emotion of the patient in order to know how to care for him or her. This innate and unique 'bridge' between the recognition of herself and her path through her healing brain injury process enables her gifts in dealing with her patients successfully and writing about it!

This book is a rare work and insight into an injured physician's mind and emotional struggle that must be read by all medical workers and patients suffering from brain injury and concussions."

Gerald Dieter Griffin, PharmD, MD, FACFE
Brigadier General, MC, USA, Retired

"A phenomenal and captivating journey into the world of TBIs from the perspective of a highly skilled physician and TBI sufferer. One's personal pilgrimage, which effectively blends real life experiences with medical science, enabling all readers to understand this challenging condition. A must read for anyone even remotely connected to someone who has a TBI or could very well suffer one from serving in our military or playing sports to riding a bicycle or tripping on a walk. Equally, it is a must read for anyone in human resources to better understand the challenges of a TBI sufferer in the workplace."

Tim A. Garrett
Retired CHRO, Honda of America Mfg., Inc.

"Dr. Gordon brings a rare combination as an author, both as a physician with deep experience in rehabilitative medicine and as someone who has personally suffered a traumatic brain injury and knows how difficult the journey to recovery can be. She also possesses an unmatched passion to help those who have also suffered a traumatic brain injury. That powerful combination of experience and true understanding has made her a leading advocate in shining the light on this major "wound of war" that has, until now, been so misunderstood. This book will speak to those in the medical profession who treat those with TBI as well as caregivers. Perhaps most important, Dr. Gordon provides hope, guidance, and light at the end of the tunnel for those that have experienced the same blackness that she herself has lived."

Justice Evelyn Lundberg Stratton, Retired
Ohio Supreme Court

"This book serves an important purpose in highlighting the persistent, serious consequences of even seemingly mild head trauma. Turn the Lights On! deserves a wide readership among sports trainers, team doctors, primary care physicians, and even neurologists. Today, many patients with chronic post concussive symptoms get "blown off" as malingerers or whiners, doing them a serious injustice. Importantly, this book provides hope that recovery is possible and resources are available to "turn on the light.""

Janet W. Bay, MD
System Vice President, Neuroscience, OhioHealth

Turn the Lights On!
A Physician's Personal Journey from the Darkness of Traumatic
Brain Injury (TBI) to Hope, Healing, and Recovery

Chrisanne Gordon, MD and Andrew Miller

Published by: Corpus Callosum Creations, Ltd.

ISBN: 978-0692999561

DEDICATION

This book is dedicated to all those whose lives have been touched by brain injuries—patients and family members alike, especially our veterans who sustain injuries in their service to our nation. Your willingness to assist in research, awareness, and recovery will ultimately change the course of medical history—from the battlefield to the playing field ... and beyond!

CONTENTS

FOREWORD

"Brain injuries don't discriminate" is a phrase that has been used quite often by a number of professional organizations who specialize in traumatic brain injury, including public safety campaigns and even the media. This statement is quite true—brain injuries can happen to anyone, at any time, and almost anywhere.

I have worked as a licensed physical therapist for almost 30 years and as a certified athletic trainer for over 16 years, and I can assure you that brain injuries don't discriminate—they can occur in sports and recreational activities, at work, driving a car, serving on active duty in the US military, and in almost any other setting or activity you can imagine.

The primary causes of brain injury in the United States are from falls, motor vehicle accidents, and being struck by or against an object (for example, during organized sports and recreational activities or due to a physical assault). Different age groups are at a higher risk for receiving a brain injury; children under the age of 14 and older adults over age 65 are at a greater risk than other age groups for brain injuries due to falls. Motor vehicle collisions are the leading cause of brain injury in children and young adults ages 5 to 24 years old (according to the Centers for Disease Control and Prevention). Brain injuries, therefore, are everyone's concern.

In the military, the causes of brain injury are quite similar to civilian (or non-military) brain injuries: falls, motor vehicle crashes, being struck by or against an object, and assaults. Traumatic brain injuries (or TBI) have drawn intense media attention in the past decade-and-a-half due to conflicts in Iraq, Afghanistan, and elsewhere. These TBIs have been labelled as the "invisible wound of war," along with post-traumatic stress disorder and other mental health consequences of combat experiences.

As increased attention has been made for these "invisible" injuries, more research has been devoted to better strategies for prevention, management, and treatment among active duty service members and veterans. The advancements in research, increased media focus, and a wealth of educational information about TBIs, particularly those that are "mild" in nature, is changing the notion that brain injuries are "invisible"—there are clinical signs (observed by health care professionals) and reported symptoms (noted by the patient or family member) that may prompt someone to seek medical care and get on the road to recovery.

For those patients with a TBI, progress can be observed as they recover physically, emotionally (or psychologically), and cognitively (e.g. thinking skills)—progress that is visible to both the patient and those who care for them. Through greater awareness, better outreach, and improved educational approaches, TBI is becoming the "visible" invisible wound. Brain injury is no longer an injury we can't "see," understand, or comprehend. This book will help you, the reader, gain a better understanding into the causes, effects, and recovery from TBI—and it will open your eyes in a new way when it comes to looking at brain injuries.

Franklin D. Roosevelt, the 32nd President of the United States, once said, "When you come to the end of your rope, tie a knot and hang on." This book, *Turn the Lights On! A Physician's Journey from the Darkness of Traumatic Brain Injury (TBI) to Hope, Healing, and Recovery,* by Dr. Chrisanne Gordon and Andrew Miller, reminds us that we must do just what President Roosevelt said—"tie a knot and hang on."

Brain injuries can result in a series of life-changing events, both for the person who sustained the injury and those who take care of them. A traumatic brain injury can impact every aspect of one's life—family, school, work, recreation and leisure, and more—and the injury can have short-lasting or longer-lasting effects on a person's physical (body), mental, emotional, and even spiritual well-being.

A brain injury is not the end—for patients, overcoming a brain injury may feel at times like the "end of your rope," but it is a process and a journey that you will learn and grow from as you receive care from a variety of health care professionals and from the support from your family and caregivers. For caregivers (which may include spouses, parents, children, co-workers, or professional caregivers), you too may often feel like you are at "the end of your rope." Please know that there is hope after a brain injury—there is always hope, progress, improvements, and, most importantly, the next chapter of your lives. I hope that you will find this book as inspiring and relevant to you as it has been for me.

Scott C. Livingston, PhD, PT, ATC
Defense and Veterans Brain Injury Center,
United States Defense Health Agency

PREFACE

I magine a room that you know like the back of your hand. A room that you designed, decorated, and have lived in for much of your life. A room that is safe and brings you comfort, a room that is truly yours. Now stand in the doorway, turn off the lights, and walk inside. At some point you will harmlessly bump into something, which at first will be more annoying than anything else, but as you continue to walk around bumping into more and more things the room will become disheveled and your frustration will build. Your instincts will eventually guide you towards the door and the comfort of the light. Yet, in this room the switch is broken and the door is shut. You try not to panic as you have many other rooms you can access, but you know that life will bring you back into this room over and over again and the struggle will ensue as you attempt to turn on the light.

This simple and alarming scenario provides a glimpse into the daily struggles of those of us living with a traumatic brain injury (TBI). Invisible tears within the very fabric of our consciousness that wreak havoc not only on our mind, body, and soul, but also on those people closest to us.

Invisible wound with many causes, a TBI does not discriminate by age, gender, ethnicity, or background. Instead, they often lay dormant for months, if not years, before taking effect. Once they do, they take hold of anyone unfortunate enough to be in their path. When present, TBI is undoubtedly one of the most devastating disorders a person and their family can face given how complex and misunderstood it is.

The scenario portrayed above was shared with me by Dr. Chrisanne Gordon, shortly after we first met in the spring of 2012. Dr. Gordon was just forming the Resurrecting Lives Foundation and my family was exploring ways in which we could do our part in supporting military veterans and their families. From the very first conversation, Dr. Gordon's passion, purity, and purpose shot across the phone like a lightning bolt energizing everyone in earshot.

It was undeniable that she was not simply looking to make a difference; she was devoted to creating a positively disruptive change in the lives of our nation's greatest heroes: our soldiers and veterans. She had the experience, the facts, and the drive; but most importantly she had the guts to put it all on the line for the greater good.

All she was missing was the public spotlight to shine on these inconvenient truths surrounding TBI and the systems tasked with their care. Truths that, if the public were given a choice about, few would find acceptable for our veterans, let alone any loved ones.

Awoken to the truth, my family and many others now stand in support of Dr. Gordon and the Resurrecting Lives Foundation in their mission to bring awareness, treatment, employment, hope, and ultimately recovery to the hundreds of thousands of military veterans returning home from Iraq and Afghanistan who suffer from TBI and post-traumatic stress disorder (PTSD).

To no one's surprise, Dr. Gordon's tenacity and charm opened one door after another, and her selfless advocacy and warrior spirit inspire everyone she meets. Whether in the halls of Congress or the boardrooms of corporate America, Dr. Gordon makes her mission clear and settles for nothing less than what our veterans deserve—peace. A peace that we owe to those who have sacrificed so very much, and a peace that is truly within our ability to give. If you agree, the question then becomes how one person, one group, or one community can make a difference in something that few can even see.

I believe it begins with the understanding that our freedom is not free, and every day that our brave men and women are deployed abroad they are doing so not only to protect our country. These heroes are doing this job for us, our values, and the freedom to live the lives we choose with the ones we love. They place duty ahead of desire and they do so for us all. Yet, when faced with repaying our debt to these men and women who may have suffered TBI or PTSD, we haven't put duty first; as a result, few veterans are provided the solutions and support they deserve. This has led to a spike in veteran homelessness, unemployment, alcoholism, and tragically, suicide ... all of which are unacceptable in this age of abundance.

I believe the solution has to be bigger than the problem, and in the case of TBI the solution rests within society itself. We must embrace a culture of positive disruption, of radical research and innovation such as Dr. Gordon represents. Because in this case, on this topic, there should be no stone left unturned, no strategy untried, and no care given without the highest consideration of what we are fighting for—our nation's future and the repayment of a debt that will never be called.

We owe it to our veterans and ourselves to stand together in the fight against TBI—to bring the injury and the injured out of the shadows and into the light. We have the power to overcome this enemy; we have the resources to improve these lives; we simply need the courage to stand up for those who stood for us and all we hold dear. Let us turn the lights on for TBI and let the light of change be everlasting.

Gregory Welteroth, Jr.

Gregory Welteroth Jr. and the Welteroth Family have been leading efforts to care for wounded veterans for years through their philanthropy and direct action. Gregory Welteroth, Jr. is the President of Gregory Welteroth Advertising.

ACKNOWLEDGMENTS

I t is with deep gratitude that I wish to acknowledge those individuals who so closely guided me during this project, especially my incredibly gifted co-writer, Andrew Miller, and my amazingly disciplined editor, Kathy Balas Lucisano. Although I just met Andrew as we began this journey together, Kathy and I have been friends since we met in first grade, though I had lost contact with her for a mere 35 years. Time and distance dissolved at her first "surprise" email correspondence, which should have been no surprise at all, given our connection. Kathy and Andrew appearing in my life at the same time made all the difference. This stroke of luck was inherited from my Irish grandfather, Neil Cronin, who first taught me that luck was *"preparation meeting opportunity."*

I want to thank my teachers, especially those in medical school, who taught me to always listen to the patient, which becomes strikingly more challenging when you become the patient.

I also must acknowledge, at the beginning of this book, and at the end of every day, my constant companions: my patients, my young athletes, and, especially, my military members, veterans, and their families who have spent countless hours telling their stories and assisting in my current understanding of this oxymoron classified as "mild" brain injury.

CHAPTER ONE

LIGHTS OUT

I was (and still am), like a nerve, like the brain, like a microprocessor, wired as an ON/OFF entity. I worked fast and furiously while awake, then slept deeply and soundly. There was no fatigue time, no depression settling in, just a hypomania that drove me to achieve the goals I'd laid out before me from intern, to resident, to successful ER doctor, to rehabilitation physician.

This was my life prior to suffering a traumatic brain injury.

"God, please do not let me wake up a quad,"—in the amount of time it took for this brief prayer, the lights went out. I'd felt a stinger, this wave like an overwhelming electrical shock, flow down my cervical nerve root—C5 to C6—and down both arms. By no means had time itself slowed, but my thoughts raced ahead of the encroaching darkness. I knew a significant amount of force had transmitted to my spine, and if I fractured my cervical spine I may well awake a quadriplegic.

Since the time I was eight years old I have been a caregiver to those around me. In my adult life as a doctor I chose to make a career out of caregiving. I lived alone. I took care of myself. It was how I operated. How would I function as a caregiver if I could no longer care for myself? If I required someone else to bathe me, feed me, and clothe me? How would I be brave enough to be at someone else's mercy? I was terrified at the prospect of accepting this as my new reality.

There wasn't a moment where the proverbial life-flashed-before-my-eyes took place since I wasn't having a near-death experience, but I did have this momentary memory that closely coincided with my potential injuries. I pictured my childhood kitchen. My mother thrust my shrieking two-day-old baby sister into my arms so she and my father could similarly shriek at one another in front of my ten-year-old brother Neil, five-year-old sister Patty, and me.

My mother, falling into what we now know as postpartum depression, ran to the bedroom to hide her tears and to avoid the rest of us for the next day and a half. Father handed me a half-empty baby bottle, left our home, and fled to the safety of his own medical practice. I stood there cradling the closest I'd come to having a child, my newborn sister, who incessantly wailed like a frightened animal.

Like most children—people in general, really—we all have our own way to cope on those occasions when life loses tranquility. Neil chilled out, sat in the high-back chair in the living room, listened to music, and rocked back and forth in a sort of rhythmic, reflective trance. My sister Patty joined in the screams of the newborn, not having developed her own coping mechanism for this situation as of yet even though she was no longer the baby of the family. At that moment I had to reach way down inside myself to engage all the survival skills I could muster—not just for myself, but for all of us—learning, at that moment in time, that my coping mechanism was to take care and take charge.

That night I served TV dinners and a warm bottle for the newborn while we all sat quietly, and unsupervised, and watched whatever tuned in on our television. While this wouldn't go down as the best care I might ever provide, it was the day I became a caregiver and never looked back. Making order out of external chaos became a way of life for me.

But I was about to have chaos within, and that is an entirely different matter.

When I came to from the blackout, I felt as if I were at the bottom of a lake, floating in the darkness and unable to see the surface. I couldn't focus my eyes; I couldn't focus my mind. It took me several minutes before even realizing that I was splayed out, flat on my back upon the floor. I didn't move because I didn't think I could; all I could do is hope that my friend, Terry, would come over and discover me as we planned to have dinner that evening.

Most Saturdays I'd rise about 6:30 a.m. and then head in to work from about 8 until 2 in the afternoon. This day was a little different though, given that it was Thanksgiving weekend. I planned on watching several key NCAA football games, plus my "baby" sister was coming into town for a visit. I'd been very excited for her visit because they were always enjoyable.

I woke to a dark November sky that invoked the feel of a fall chill and this sense of foreboding, which left a wariness in the pit of my stomach. Even ABC sports reporter Keith Jackson commented on how a 20-mph wind was keeping things cool all the way down in Florida, where he'd been calling one of the several NCAA games I'd been looking forward to.

I'd thought the premonition had been answered after a call came through from my boyfriend, who had been in a fender bender that morning. Both cars were damaged but no injuries to report. As such, the edginess I'd felt upon arising that morning dissipated and I embraced my afternoon with vigor, looking forward once again to watching first-ranked University of Florida play second-ranked Florida State University while decorating the house for Christmas. (This game was particularly important to me as it would decide who my team, the Notre Dame Fighting Irish, could play on New Year's Day if the Irish managed to beat USC that evening. At this point, Notre Dame had beaten USC 11 years straight and under Lou Holtz had no intention of losing this year either.)

As the last seconds of the first half ticked down, University of Florida's head coach, Steve Spurrier (a favorite of mine both as a Heisman Trophy winning All-American quarterback who went on to the NFL and then as a coach), looked forward to the second half when the Gators would no longer have the wind in their face. Spurrier hoped that his number-one offense in the league could overcome the number-one defense of Florida State with a little help from Mother Nature. At the half, though, Florida State led 17 to 14. Unfortunately, fate wasn't on the side of the University of Florida that day, either, as they would fall to Florida State in this season-ending matchup.

I had no reason to know in those final seconds before halftime that the Gators weren't the only ones headed for a loss. Fortunately, for them, redemption wouldn't be far off. The loss meant the

Gators got a chance for a rematch against the Seminoles at that year's Sugar Bowl, which the University of Florida won, securing the South Eastern Conference championship.

My loss-turned-victory would take a lot longer than theirs. For me the last thing I would read and remember clearly for about the next four months was that 17-to-14 half-time score. Perhaps the singular silver lining to come of my injury was not remembering Notre Dame's defeat that night at the hands of USC, breaking their 11-year winning streak.

Holidays at my house were never celebrated with significant gusto, particularly because I lived alone and I was a workaholic. Home décor took a back seat to taking care of patients and reading up on the latest medical literature. However, with my baby sister visiting soon, I'd pulled several boxes of Christmas decorations, place settings, and the like from the basement crawlspace of my two-story suburban Ohio home. My usual idea of Christmas decorations included a small fake tree and enough ornaments to fill an hour of my time. As I pulled the boxes marked *holidays* from the crawlspace I looked in each one to determine if I wanted to use what was inside or to put it back for another year. When I came to the heavy-duty 12 place settings of Christmas china I decided that even with my sister in town, we were sticking with what was already in the cupboards. There was no way I felt like carrying about 70 pounds of china upstairs for one meal.

The basement had a low-pile carpet throughout, except for near the entrance of the crawlspace, which was polished concrete. In order to assess what would stay and what would go I'd pulled the boxes out onto the carpet. In returning them to their storage place I had to use every bit of my 120-pound frame to push that

70-pound box of china back into the crawlspace. I'd put in motion a test of physics I was sure to lose. Friction between the box and carpet gave way to the smooth, slick concrete. A masonry wall surrounded the miniature crawlspace door. As the box crossed the threshold of resistance to involuntary sliding, my momentum overwhelmed my control and I very literally hit a brick wall.

At that exact moment I knew this was unlike any other injury I'd experienced in my life. I was losing consciousness, rapidly, and I fought to stay awake but it was useless. To this day I'm not sure how long I was unconscious, but I remember regaining consciousness only to realize I couldn't feel my right arm or leg, and I was afraid to even attempt to move for at least another 10 or 20 minutes. I was overwhelmed with the situation and concerned that if I had broken my neck I might do further damage. Eventually, after many minutes, I decided I needed to know if I could move even a little. I felt a serious, worrisome brain-to-body disconnect. In my mind my thoughts about moving carried on as if everything was normal, but in reality my limbs moved very slowly, ignoring my mind's commands. The physician in me wanted to understand but I couldn't muster one intelligent thought as to what was happening. My inner patient deemed it wise to find help.

While I hoped I'd be found sooner than later by Terry, there was no guarantee. I felt trapped in the basement and very alone, not even a pet in the house to come to my side. The TV remained on in the finished part of the basement as my only connection to the outside world, and as the only basis for guessing how long I'd been immobile. I waited another two hours, judging by the advancement of the football games, praying that Terry or my sister would come over and find me. I'd seen people in my rehabilitation work who were able to get themselves up and walk away after an injury like this and then they sneeze or roll over in their sleep (or something similarly insignificant that becomes extremely significant)—just enough to dislodge the spine, leaving them paralyzed or worse. Even though I was terrified of this becoming my reality, I knew I needed to get to medical help, get x-rayed, and get treatment. None of that was going to happen as long as I lay alone on the cold cement floor of that crawlspace.

I hesitantly began to move. My head hurt so much when I attempted to lift it that I opted to crawl slowly across the room to the staircase, and then even more slowly up the half-flight of stairs out of the basement and into the kitchen. By my best estimate it was about 4:30 p.m. at this point; the Florida—Florida State game had started at noon. I still could not stand, so I dragged my numb body to a chair near the phone and pulled myself up. I grabbed hold of the cordless phone. I remember staring at the phone and thinking I could do something with it to get help, but how I should use it wouldn't register in my mind. I stared but never saw any buttons or numbers for it appeared as a blank slate before my eyes.

Holding this potentially lifesaving tool in my uncooperative hands, I waited for my memory to clear up enough to remember what I was supposed to do with it. I had no idea—what it was or how to use it. I remember staring at it, praying some saving revelation would come to me, but nothing did. I put it down, carefully, as if I might remember how to save myself with it at any moment. That moment never came. After several more minutes of frustration, I crawled to the front door of the house and laid myself there, crumpled on the floor like a sack of laundry waiting to be taken to the cleaners. Night fell and the house became darker while my last remaining hope, for my friend to arrive and find me there, became a far-off possibility.

Some seemingly long period of time later, Terry arrived, although this wasn't quite the rescue I'd hoped for. At first, Terry thought I was playing a joke. As in many cases of traumatic brain injury (TBI), the accident hadn't gashed my head open so there was no blood, and although I had a raised welt, it was obscured by my hair. Like many other victims of TBI, a lack of external trauma made my potential rescue more difficult. I continued to lie still there on the floor. My head throbbed. When I moved, I feared paralysis. I couldn't hear very well because everything came through as if it were being spoken through a pillow. My eyes remained out of focus; the darkness had helped downplay this and even seemed to calm some of my anxiety. Now, however, the foyer lights had been turned on and my ears seemed bombarded with noise from Terry requesting me to stop "playing around."

To be fair, many people who suffer a TBI suffer this indignity as well, with well-intentioned rescuers who first assume they are fooling around, drunk, or possibly on drugs. The similarities between TBI symptoms and substance abuse behaviors are striking.

The irony of the situation wasn't completely lost on me. My boyfriend had been the one in an auto accident that very day while I was just decorating my own home and watching a game on TV. It was a bitter pill to swallow that I was now the one in the care of a friend, somewhat more than an acquaintance, who could not recognize the seriousness of my situation.

Using what strength I had, I managed to pull myself up. I uttered some garbled words while I stood on wobbly legs, hoping to be understood.

"ER" is what I hoped had come out of my mouth, then the word "concussion," but given that my request was met with a blank stare, or so it seemed, I realized there was a "glitch" in my communication skills. Actually, I wasn't sure I understood what I had said, so I tried again while Terry tried again to stop my "putting on an act." Eventually I thought to use the pen and pad of paper lying on a shelf next to me. I scratched out the letters "E R!" I may not have remembered what to do with the phone, but I had been writing scripts for years, and paper and pen came right back to me, thankfully.

Terry got it this time and within the hour we were at the emergency room.

As we'll dive into more deeply later in this book, thanks to specialists and researchers such as Kalev Freeman, MD, PhD, who runs the Trauma Physiology Lab at the University of Vermont, focused on studying, in his words, "the fundamental vascular biology changes that occur following trauma," we know that the myth that states an injury only occurs if there has been a loss of consciousness is untrue. Even without a blatant, visible trauma such as a witnessed black-out or physical head wound, a cranial impact of any severity can lead to a TBI. Even more surprising is what we've learned regarding shockwaves, which can cause injury without obvious physical contact.

What I did not realize at that time was that I entered a sort of *boot-camp* for brain recovery. I had worked in the TBI rehabilitation services during my residency, and I had indeed been fascinated by the brain's ability to recover because it does so in such dramatic fashion. The brain doesn't gradually get better. It improves in chunks—either information or activity—and it does so in a way that all bystanders can witness the improvement.

When a patient's brain is chaotic, as my brain now was, how can there be survival? I barely made it to the ER, and then only because of the eventual actions of my friend, my rescuer. What about our military members who suffer brain injuries by improvised explosive devices (IEDs)? There is carnage, death, fire—destruction all around. How do these brave, brain-battered military members manage to reach safety while protecting their comrades in battle? These were questions I would pursue in the decade following my own recovery as I read about the 450,000 young men and women who served in the wars in Iraq and Afghanistan and suffered from brain injuries.[1] I would think back to the first 72 hours surrounding my battle with a brick wall and think: "How did they survive?"

Brain injuries also occur for our athletes, who suffer blow upon blow, from youth leagues up to the professionals, and are told to get back in the game. Youth sports are growing more similar to adult amateur and professional leagues, becoming more and more competitive and tasking young bodies to their limits. Even if an athlete is advised to leave the field of play, many won't because of the ever-increasing performance baseline required to remain a viable player in these highly competitive activities.

Add to that the fact that athletics are seen as a potential gateway out of poverty, both in the United States and in many other developed and developing nations, the same way military service is. For poor youth suffering a TBI, this reality means they will not only suffer the injury itself, but likely will also not have the means to afford treatment or other support for symptoms such as memory loss, depression, anxiety, decreased reaction time and dexterity, loss of balance, and hearing and vision problems. Ex-NFL running back and Ohio State University 2001 MVP Jonathan Wells confirmed that football is a way to improve your life and the life of your family. He is now part of the legal proceedings against the NFL for brain injuries sustained during his professional career. "I can remember many times while playing in the NFL where I took a hit and saw stars, but I didn't report the injury because missed playing time can lead to being unemployed," Wells stated. "So I learned early on how to get back into the huddle no matter what."

Traumatic brain injury is now known to be cumulative as well. The best predictor of a brain injury is having a previous brain injury, because with each one suffered, the individual loses some level of balance, depth perception, and spatial comprehension—all of which makes them more vulnerable to another TBI.

In the *Frontline* investigative report, "League of Denial: The NFL's Concussion Crisis,"[2] Robert Stern, PhD, Neuropsychologist at Boston University, said, "In football, one has to expect that almost every play of every game and every practice, they're going to be hitting their heads against each other. That's the nature of the game. Those things seem to happen around 1,000 to 1,500 times a year. Each time that happens, it's around 20G or more. That's the equivalent of driving a car at 35 miles per hour into a brick wall 1,000 to 1,500 times per year."

As discussed in that *Frontline* report, documents obtained by the lawyer Bob Fitzsimmons for retired NFL player "Iron" Mike Webster show that even research by NFL doctors had recorded that correlation: "The NFL acknowledges that repetitive trauma to the head in football can cause a permanent disabling injury to the brain." Due to research such as this we are now aware that repetition of upper body, and in particular head-first hits, experienced in full-contact sports or battlefield conditions are creating chronic brain injuries that only intensify over time. In North America alone the Centers for Disease Control (CDC) reported a 50 percent increase in emergency room visits or hospitalization for TBI, from 1.6 million in 2007 to 2.8 million—or one in every 50 ER visits—in 2013, the most recent year for which comprehensive figures are available.[3] That means that for every one of these TBI cases, that subset of society has then increased their chances of suffering future brain injuries, heightening the chance of needing costly long-term care. This is a cost not just tied up in medical bills but with significant social ramifications as well, including higher rates of addiction, unemployment, homelessness, and suicide.[4] TBI is also associated with a higher risk of incarceration.

This isn't just an American phenomenon either. Through my work with the Resurrecting Lives Foundation, a non-profit I founded to increase awareness and support for our veterans who suffer from TBI/PTSD, I've had the opportunity to discuss TBI statistics and research with a global community of doctors. Both in the United Kingdom and in Australia, military members have suffered from TBI and are now facing sequellae secondary to those injuries including seizures, depression, and long-term possibilities of Parkinson's and Alzheimer's.

According to a 2012 article in *The Lancet Neurology* journal, TBI is even more prevalent in underprivileged nations than in wealthier nations such as North America and Europe—where it is estimated that between 150—300 cases per 100,000 residents are reported per year.[5] Across Europe, hospitals are experiencing a rate of over 200 TBI cases per 100,000 people annually, with an average in-hospital fatality rate of 2 to 3 percent. In the United States the fatality rate is estimated closer to 6 percent according to *The Lancet Neurology*. The editors called for greater investment in understanding how to treat these injuries and provide ongoing post-trauma care due to the increased risk factors mentioned earlier, as well as increased risks for dementia and chronic traumatic encephalopathy (CTE). It is *The Lancet Neurology's* belief that without significant investment, TBI could become the third leading cause globally of disability and death by 2020.

Ongoing research around TBI and the NFL has found that 42.5 percent of the 40 retired NFL players studied by Francis X. Conidi, DO, at the Florida Center for Headache and Sports Neurology, suffered from TBI. During the 2016 American Academy of Neurology's annual meeting, Conidi reported that the study was "one of the first to demonstrate significant objective evidence for TBI in former players … we found that longer careers placed the athletes at a higher risk of TBI."[6]

Speaking personally, prior to my injury I regularly worked 24- to 36-hour shifts. If you round that out it averages about 17 hours of work per day, six out of seven days a week. Outside of office work I'd exercise, eat, and dig back into continuing my lifelong passion for learning new medical technologies and protocols. Medicine and caring for my patients was all I knew and all I wanted to do. For two years after my injury I struggled to get back to even a 10-hour work day. On top of that, any joy I'd felt for taking care of my patients had disappeared during this period. I no longer thrived on the sort of chaos and constant flow of patients I had previously. Instead I required a calm, organized, and quiet surrounding to function. I even required special incandescent lighting that could be dimmed to prevent me from feeling overwhelmed by my senses.

My once near-photographic memory never returned, the TBI leaving me struggling even to remember my patients' names. Since the brain injury, I often resorted to using clichés such as *Sweetie* or *Dear* for fear of saying the wrong name. For the first time in my life I required patients and coworkers to speak slowly to me so I could process what was being said. I would ask them to write it down or I would never remember it on my own otherwise.

This is a similar story shared by so many people who have suffered from TBI. As reported in the *Frontline* episode on concussion in the NFL, former Pittsburgh Steeler star Webster had found himself homeless. He had been arrested for forging 19 methylphenidate prescriptions, which according to Webster's son Colin, was the only thing that kept him able to function. Methylphenidate, a drug meant to jump start the brain, helped him feel more normal.

Colin went on to describe several episodes with his father, including how, "He would forget, you know, which way the grocery store was, which way it was to go home. He was—he actually—he broke down in tears in front of me a couple of times because he couldn't get his thoughts together and he couldn't keep them in order."

Like so many of the heroes I've worked with who have also suffered TBI, I felt a great deal of shame admitting to these changes in myself. Iron Mike's widow described a time where he destroyed all of his football memorabilia out of anger over what he'd been reduced to—telling a fan who recognized him on the street, who'd asked if he was indeed Iron Mike, "I used to be."

Who I used to be was an intensely left-brained person of science, logic, and study. Unlike Iron Mike and so many others, though, I have been fortunate to have the benefit of more rehabilitation than most people suffering TBI. I have since begun to learn to enjoy my right brain, my center of creativity, and embrace it as I never had before. Though I miss my left brain daily my "used to be" state is not the entirety of my identity.

What this injury and rehabilitation has given me is a new approach to life, including this mission to change the way our veterans, and anyone else suffering the debilitating effects of TBI, are rehabilitated, cared for over the long term, and reintegrated into society. In that regard there is a much brighter silver lining to my accident than just missing the opportunity to form a memory of my Fighting Irish losing to USC that year. Instead, I'm embracing this new mission in life I feel called to complete, and I'm fired up and ready to go.

HOO-AH! OO-RAH!

CHAPTER TWO

NO LIGHT ON THE BOTTOM OF THE SEA

By the time I arrived at the ER I struggled with many of the hallmark traits of TBI. I suffered from photophobia, literally translated as the fear of light. People who suffer a brain injury often have increased light sensitivity, and in fact have difficulties with headaches and dizziness from light exposure. The fluorescent light in the ER overwhelmed me and kept me from processing anything visually. My world looked like a Monet painting, speckles of color without definition. This was without the benefit that comes with a real Monet hanging in a gallery where you can choose to look away and once again see the world in all its clarity. There was a darkness surrounding all these bursts of colors as well. I was left with the foggy view anyone who has dived deep into the ocean is aware of, the distorted beam of light from the sun refracting onto the water's surface above, creating a vignette on the periphery. It was late November. It was 5 p.m. and dark outside, and I was wearing my sunglasses and still covering my eyes with my hands.

The photophobia would've been enough alone but its disorienting effect had increased my anxiety and made my heart race, adding to a feeling of dizziness and being lightheaded. Anxiety bore out not just as stress but also as an emotional lability, where I oscillated back and forth between laughing and crying, unable to stabilize my emotions as if they were merely another biological reaction taking place and not any sort of social construct brought forward by either humor or depressing news. This trait initially gave Terry the erroneous conclusion that for some strange reason, I was "faking."

I was certain I was bleeding into my brain due to the severity of the headache and my utter lack of balance. I walked slowly and was extremely uncoordinated. I wasn't even quite certain how to use the stool to boost myself onto the gurney for examination. All of these symptoms were progressively getting worse, not better, which further increased my fears and anxiety about what was to become of me.

Terry had delivered me to an excellent rural hospital where I was currently on staff, knowing that my good friend and ER staff director, Ralph Peters, MD, would be available for consultation. Fortunately he was on hand, and when he entered the room one of the few clear memories I have through the thick fog of that day was his impression of my situation, particularly how clearly concerned he was. I can't remember the intake evaluation or whether I had a long or short wait before being brought into the examination area. I can't remember if Terry waited for me in the waiting room or was there with me in the examination room. I just remember Dr. Peters acting swiftly yet gently in my seemingly slow-motion world.

Even this far removed from the day, having the benefit of having had conversations with friends and family about it, I'm surprised by how little I'm able to recall of it on my own. By the time we made it to the ER I was barely able to speak, and the presence of so many able people around me made me feel that much more impaired.

For most injured individuals, an ER staff has at best an hour to complete their evaluation and recommendation before having to move on to the next case, particularly in more urban trauma units, so being at a rural community hospital where I worked served me well. In particular, being surrounded by ER personnel whom I considered my friends and colleagues was especially helpful to my case. There wasn't a moment that they thought I was just joking or faking. For a patient with a TBI, this is a huge plus. Seeing someone who knew you pre-injury truly assists the medical assessment.

Likewise, they knew this wasn't due to drug abuse nor alcohol. In my four-year emergency physician position, I became very aware of how easy it can be to confuse a TBI patient with someone under the influence or overdosed—and this is getting worse as the drug abuse epidemic grows. Regardless, ER doctors are trained to take concussion situations seriously, as there may well be life-or-death consequences associated with whatever caused the blackout. ER staff are well aware that even providing a high level of care could still lead to further deterioration hours or days after the injury event.

Completing a neurological check is not easy, and with the current research being done on TBIs we're finding out that what we once believed to be tried and true tests can be anything but. For example, when I suffered my TBI a computerized axial tomography (CAT/CT) scan was standard procedure. A CT scan works by x-raying the body in a 360-degree capture and then processing the image through a computer, allowing the physician to see a series of slices, similar to how you might pull out individual slices of a loaf of bread. The scan generally shows whether or not an organ appears to be functioning as normal or has suffered some sort of trauma. For example, a CT scan is able to show bleeding of the brain, such as from an aneurysm, but we now know the CT scan is not very effective for observing brain injuries that do not create a bleeding or significant bruising effect on the brain. Eventually a combination CT scan and magnetic resonance imaging (MRI) test was added to the protocol for diagnosing patients suspected of a TBI. While the MRI provides an even greater level of brain tissue detail than a CT scan, it still isn't perfect. An MRI can see more minute changes in the brain structure than a CT scan is able, and the technology keeps improving. Unfortunately, neither of these highly sophisticated methods were able to diagnose what had happened to me. By this time, I was aphasic, that is, unable to speak. I had no feeling on the right side of my body. My studies, including an x-ray of my cervical spine, were normal. I, however, was not going to be "normal" ever again.

Since the time of my TBI we've learned that in many cases, particularly in the case of a mild TBI, neither a CT scan nor an MRI will provide physicians with the information they need to correctly diagnose the injury. This alone is a troubling fact given that these tests are the basis of the current protocol for people coming to the ER complaining of a potential concussion or other brain injury. With additional funding for research, and with the advent of TBI registries, I hope we may soon develop protocols or discover newer diagnostic tools.

Researchers Chris Hagen, PhD, Danese Malkmus, MA, and Patricia Durham, MA, working in the 1970s for the Rancho Los Amigos Hospital in Downey, California developed the Rancho Los Amigos Levels of Cognitive Functioning Scale,*[7] referred to often as the Rancho scale, RLAS, or LOCF. This scale rates a patient's cognitive function from *Level I—No Response: Total Assistance,* to *Level X—Purposeful, Appropriate: Modified Independent.* When I arrived at the ER I was what we now may judge as *Level V—Confused, Inappropriate Non-Agitated: Maximal Assistance.* However, even to this day making an assessment based on this soundly researched scale is more for the diagnosis of severe or moderate TBI, but not mild TBI. The diagnostic protocols for mild TBI are still being worked out.

Dr. Peters stated that my studies were normal. I believe I started to cry because it seemed impossible to me. Even more seemingly impossible was that, even in my current state, I was being sent home with a friend and a standard "concussion" checklist that most people are at least aware of, if not familiar with. It is the instruction sheet requiring the concussed person be awakened every hour to check and make sure they know what time it is and where they are, etc. Unable to express myself intelligibly, I felt sheer panic over the idea that I was being put back into the

---

* See Resources for full text of current scale.

care of my friend. The same friend who originally thought I was making this all up as a joke, and now had been told everything is normal according to the tests. Although I recognized that I was not Terry's responsibility, I felt a sinking feeling that there was no chance she would wake me up per the doctor's orders, and I was certain I'd hemorrhage in the middle of the night and be severely impaired. The thought of dying was not yet a reality for me; that would come a few weeks later.

To put this further into perspective, according to a peer-reviewed study completed by Dr. Martina Stippler, Assistant Professor of Neurological Surgery, Director of Neurotrauma at the University of New Mexico, "routine follow-up CT scans rarely alter treatment for patients with complicated mild TBI."[8] Stippler questions the utility of these CT scans as they only seem to alter treatment if hemorrhaging occurs, implying that they are meaningless in cases like mine. Adding to this, the Rancho Scale level of cognition at which I was functioning (Level V) meant Dr. Peters and the other staffers, as well as Terry, witnessed all of the following: my lack of orientation, unsustainable attention, inability to take in new information or recall any sort of recent memories, and agitation to several external stimulants such as light and noise. I was able to provide some verbalization of my situation and perform simple tasks as long as I received enough prompting, but without cues from others I was pretty helpless. A diagnosis of Level V symptoms means that I was in need of *maximum assistance*. Even if I had cleared to a Level VI I would still have required what Rancho dictates as *moderate assistance*—so in no way did I believe that being sent home fit any of this diagnosis given that the one thing I did know was I'd have to care for myself there. So, being the patient rather than the physician truly put me in a very anxious state, with my perception of my current situation skewed by my sudden disabilities. My scans were normal; my vitals were normal; my physical well-being was not in question. Of course I should be discharged, but, for the first time in my life since I was eight years old and handed my baby sister, I felt that I was not that capable of caring for myself. Luckily, I would be proven wrong.

I attempted to mouth something about how concerned I was, but the best I could do was to try and grab the doctor's arm, as if to beg him to admit me, but I was unable to communicate that concern. Before sending me on my way, Dr. Peters notified a neurosurgeon who I knew and trusted who said she would be on call, not far from my house, in case any difficulties arose over night. This was a glimmer of hope for me were the worst to come over the next eight to ten hours.

Here's the difficulty of the concussion protocol and being released from the ER that all too many families are familiar with: an individual with a TBI may look completely normal but that doesn't mean they can follow through with ER instructions, or even understand them in many situations. A TBI patient is completely at the mercy of their caregiver. A brain injury doesn't just impact the injured, it becomes a family issue, and sometimes a community issue because it is always family or friends left to care for all but the most severe TBI patients. In one of the support groups I take part in locally (the TBI Think Tank) I sit in conversation with family members of TBI patients to better understand the challenges faced not only by the patient, but by their caregivers.

One mother I've worked with said that she carries a great deal of guilt over what she describes as her constant nagging of her son who suffered multiple TBI through athletics. He's become socially isolated because his friends found it too difficult to include him in their activities due to his struggle to remember what he is doing, and some of his behaviors. She has learned over time that repeated, gentle requests are more effective than statements—such as the difference between the request, "Did you happen to take out the trash?" versus the demand, "Take out the trash now." For her son, a demand is interpreted by his brain as a sort of challenge that overwhelms him, leaving him unable to react. Another mother in the group said that she sometimes wishes her son would wear a tee shirt announcing his TBI because just to look at him he seems like a completely normal young man, but to interact with him you notice that he is extremely explicit and agitated, likely due to frontal lobe damage—the part of the brain that tends to act as a social filter. For this reason, like so many other sufferers of TBI, her son, too, is also very socially isolated. Her greatest frustration so far has been how little it seems that her son's health care providers understand about the stages of recovery from TBI. Indeed, despite the growing traumatic brain injury epidemic worldwide, only 8 to 10 percent of health care providers are skilled in the proper diagnosis and treatment.

Marine Sgt. Christopher Lawrence's story is a prime example of how difficult it can be to detect TBI in a young, physically fit veteran. Lawrence, who lost his right leg below the knee, and lost use of his left arm in an IED explosion while the bridge he was crossing in Iraq was blown up, is the perfect case in point. Standing 6'2" tall, with a toned physique and an aura of leadership and strength, no one would suspect he had any injuries, let alone a TBI. However, common sense would dictate that any explosion forceful enough to blow off limbs would definitely affect brain function. Lawrence, who speaks with a resonating voice that even James Earl Jones may envy, explains this public misconception in his interview during the filming of the 2012 documentary, *Operation Resurrection*.[9] As Lawrence points to his skull and crossbones prosthetic on his right leg, he admits that "This was nothing. I was up and walking around in two days with my new prosthetic. It took over a year for me to be able to balance my checkbook."

The recovery from physical injuries to our bodies, such as broken arms or torn muscles, is often rooted in repetitive exercises which result in minor improvements each time they are completed. However, with brain injuries the recovery requires repetitive exercises and generally shows no minor improvements, no half-steps. There are only seemingly giant leaps at unpredictable timeframes, such as is the case of a certain young man injured in a motor vehicle accident. Following a head-on collision in his car at the age of 17, he was unable to speak—among many other issues. Then, seemingly out of nowhere, he awoke one morning and began speaking complete and coherent sentences. I'll dive deeper into this phenomenon later in the book, but this is a pearl of wisdom that many physicians and caregivers remain ignorant of—finding some way to continue to exercise the brain even if it seems like it has no impact, because eventually a connection will be made. Just like a light bulb turning on when the circuit is made whole again by flipping a switch, the electricity will flow.

This day, of turning the switch and speaking freely, was still some ways away for me. While riding in the car on my way home, I erroneously believed I would be "all better" in a day or two. By the time I arrived it was late, so Terry helped me to get situated for bed and offered to stay over. Anticipating Terry not waking up in order to check on me each hour of the night as prescribed by my doctor, I spent 10 minutes or more setting my alarm clock to wake me, I hoped, one hour later. My blurred vision and slow reaction time made it nearly impossible to stop the digital numbers whizzing by in time, but eventually I managed. Not unlike my earlier experience with the phone, seemingly simple technologies felt beyond my capability. As suspected, when that first alarm bell rang I woke to find that Terry had at least stayed in the house with me but was sleeping soundly. This made me wonder how more people like me don't end up deteriorating from this kind of injury; and I don't mean just from some sort of negligence. For those individuals who may not have a caregiver to count on at all, the situation can be very dangerous. Perhaps the caregiver may work nights, etc., and not be able to afford time off—the mathematics of lower income and fewer resources tend to add up to potential tragedy.

After another 10- to 15-minute struggle to set the alarm for the next hour, I went back to sleep and repeated this dance a few more times before giving up. I was too groggy to continue caring and too frustrated with my inability to work this simple device to want to try again. As long as I was still breathing I figured I was OK enough. Thank God by morning I did, in fact, wake up, but my brain was far from awake, and still several weeks from awakening.

CHAPTER THREE

WHEN WILL I SEE THE LIGHT

Dark is dark, both literally and metaphorically, and all the TBI patients I've ever talked to can relate to this: the darkness of blurred vision; the darkness of no longer understanding myself or the world I'm living in; the ironic need for darkness because the light is too much stimulation for my disconnected circuits to stand.

The day after my accident I awoke from the four or so hours of sleep I'd managed once my will to reset my hourly alarm had vanished. It was good to know I was still alive, but depressing that the grogginess remained, that my speech was still impaired, and that it felt impossible to focus on anything.

In a study of Alabama National Guard veterans returning from active duty in Afghanistan and Iraq, researcher Norman Keltner, EdD, RN, CRNP, found that TBI caused by the concussive forces of blasts such as IED explosions caused many of these service members to endure this metaphorical darkness as well, noting memory loss and cognitive difficulties, low attention span, fatigue, and depression.[10] An additional study funded by the National Institute of Health (NIH) conducted by several members of the Department of Neurology, University Hospital of Zurich, Switzerland, found that 95 percent of patients with moderate to severe TBI had abnormally low levels of hypocretin, which has been found to be the cause of chronic drowsiness and severe narcolepsy, with additional links to Parkinson's disease and other disorders.[11] According to the report, "Chronic excessive daytime sleepiness is a major disabling symptom for many TBI patients." The report further noted connections of TBI to sleep-wake disturbances and its impact on cognition, attention, fatigue, and depression.

In an interview with Staff Sgt. Curtis Armstrong, a veteran of Operation Iraqi Freedom, who joined the US Army just before the 9/11 terrorist attacks in 2001 working as a military police officer, he explained that his TBI occurred following a mortar attack on his base where he had been responsible for helping to train Iraqi police officers.

"Our job was basically to police Baghdad. We weren't a forward operating base but, instead, we were an academy where we were training Iraqi police officers for minor security assignments and we were running security patrols in Baghdad. We had some perimeter defenses like concrete walls and guard towers, but we were also sort of an easy target because this was a hot zone near the Ministry of Oil and Ministry of Interior and so on; so we had mortar attacks every couple days.

"I was in a guard tower with two Iraqi police officers when one of these mortar attacks launched and I was leaning over the edge to see if my buddy's tower had been hit when a mortar hit at the base of my tower. Now, a mortar blast explodes upward in a V-shape so it was like I'd been hit full on by a linebacker. I couldn't see anything and I couldn't hear. I'd been knocked over and I thought, wow, I was just in the blast, and I was touching my face and all over to make sure I wasn't ripped to shreds.

"Shortly after, someone came to check on us and they made me come down from the tower to go to the small medical building we had on site."

At this point, Armstrong apologized for getting off track, taking a moment to recollect his thoughts and explaining how he has difficulty maintaining his train of thought. This led to his explaining that early on after the injury he was prescribed a drug often used to treat ADHD. He said it helped him significantly with his anxiety and some other PTSD-related symptoms, but only served to further mask the underlying TBI.

"In the medical building I was prescribed a steroid for my ears and some ibuprofen. I wasn't noticing anything specific but it was clear that I wasn't sleeping well and I noticed that everyone seemed moody and I was fatigued, but during that time deployed you're going through so many changes that it's hard to say what's going on. So when I got back and I had headaches and the light bothered me and everything, everyone just said, 'Oh, it's PTSD.' My ability to remember stuff was scary. I couldn't remember what happened last week, and you get frustrated and then people say you're just depressed."

After this tour, Armstrong returned to the US to continue his service as an army recruiter in Mansfield, Ohio.

"With a TBI, one thing is that it can be hard to describe what's happening to yourself, much less anyone else. And your higher ups are just soldiers too. They're not doctors and they don't want to hear that you're less than capable. Like, if I came back missing an arm or something it is easy to diagnose and know how to treat—but not with TBI. And at the time everything was PTSD. It was in the media a lot so if your memory was a little off, or you're having anxiety, can't sleep—whatever—you have PTSD and just need a little time off."

Eventually Armstrong said he was sent to Walter Reed along with several of his fellow recruiters who had been complaining about the same sorts of issues.

"At first I thought maybe it was as much that our higher ups wanted to make sure we weren't making things up. But then, at Walter Reed they spent a little time with us. We were only there like two or three days, and the doctors there said, 'Well this seems like PTSD, but there's more to it that you should probably get checked out.' And I thought, well, I don't have access to any other way to get these other things checked out. It was like having a doctor tell you they found cancer but they wouldn't recommend a treatment, instead I had to find that on my own," Armstrong said.

These days Armstrong lives close to his parents in Michigan but still returns to Ohio to visit his children. He explained that the travel is difficult, and because of his issues with focus he has to rely heavily on the GPS system to navigate back and forth between the states.

"For now my kids like my company because my brain is in some ways more like a kid: scattered and unfocused," Armstrong said. "I'm not so sure they'll always think it's fun though."

* * *

My nurse friend, Karen, was in town for a visit from Florida, and I'd been looking forward to having Sunday brunch with her for several weeks. Even though I'd had such a restless night and was not by any means feeling myself, I was determined to shake off my grogginess and see my friend. I remember it taking an extraordinary amount of time to get ready. Instead of my usual 40-minute routine I spent at least two hours getting myself groomed and dressed. It was during this process I realized there would be no way I could drive myself to Bob Evans to meet her. Terry actually expressed some concern at my condition and offered to drive me, an inclination I wisely heeded. If there was concern, I must have been acting strangely.

Topographical disorientation, sometimes referred to as topographagnosia, is caused by a brain injury affecting the special processing centers, resulting in an incapacity to position oneself in one's surroundings. Watching any sort of high-impact sports will eventually give a glimpse into what this looks like—such as watching films of an NFL football player. After being concussed, you can see it in him as he's moved off the field, or placed back to the line of scrimmage. If not taken out of the game, this same player will often fumble, miss a tackle, or otherwise make a mistake that he would not have ordinarily made in his pre-concussed condition. This may be a very brief moment in time when considering athletics, but with repetition the results may mean more significant damage leading to the disorientation becoming both more debilitating and potentially permanent. Similarly, when you apply this to the battlefield you can imagine how quickly this can become a serious liability.

Public records obtained from US Veterans Affairs (VA) by some of the soldiers who have appealed to the agency for "Entitlement to service connection for residuals of a traumatic brain injury (TBI)," have reported symptoms of topographagnosia, stating that they no longer had a "sense of direction" and became easily confused about where they were or where they were going (including but not limited to Docket No. 09-20 112[12]). As of January 16, 2014, the VA has approved five secondary service conditions presumed to be connected with TBI that generally fall under the categories of physical and mental impairment. However, the VA is explicit that a soldier who suffers from Parkinson's disease, unprovoked seizures, dementia, depression, or diseases of hormone deficiency after their service, but who did not receive a diagnosis of a TBI when it occurred, are still not going to be presumed to have had a TBI that elicited these symptoms. This means that many of our veterans will be denied services because "lay evidence" (such as topographagnosia, general depression, confusion, etc.) is not "sufficient evidence to demonstrate that a TBI occurred in service."* Still, this is an encouraging move toward better brain assessment and care.

The danger is obvious when considering what this type of confusion can mean to military personnel in battle, but what we take for granted in our day-to-day life can have wide implications as well. For me these implications have become a fixture in my life, which first became apparent when Terry dropped me off at Bob Evans.

At the restaurant Terry pulled into the lot and found an empty space on the side of the building, parking long enough

---

* See Resources for the official VA definition of Traumatic Brain Injury.

to wish me well and let me out. As I started walking toward the building I turned to see Terry wave goodbye, in slow motion, only to realize I didn't know where the front door was. I spent the next 20 minutes or so wandering to and fro, back and forth around the building and parking lot, trying to find the front door. There were moments when I had to remind myself that I was looking for the front door. When I finally made it inside, Karen was there, but somewhat horrified by how I was acting. She's a great nurse, and through all of my struggle to converse with her, even just to keep conscious of what was going on, she knew I needed help and called Terry to return for me.

The entire rest of that day is a loss for me. I only remember waking up, or maybe a better term would be to say coming to, back in my house. I had no idea how I'd gotten there. I tried to sleep it off but I was feeling over-stimulated by everything. I shut out all the light I could in my bedroom and made it completely silent. Once again I was on my own. So I struggled with the alarm clock to wake every four hours to make sure I was still alive.

For as confused and upsetting as the day before had been, this day, the one I'd hoped to have awoken feeling somewhat back to normal, proved to be an even more stressful day as the reality of my situation hit me hard. The only functions my body seemed willing to continue to abide by were breathing, eating, and sleeping—and even that seemed beyond my ability to comprehend. Nothing else worked. It was as if my brain had been wiped clean without even the luxury of a basic sort of operating system being reinstalled. The darkness I felt from having so much taken from me was, as I said, one part of the darkness; but the darkness I craved—lying motionless in a silent and dark room—was the only space I could find comfort in, at least until my circuits kicked in and my brain could once again light up.

Monday morning came and I took a taxi cab to work and caught a ride home from a colleague. I wasn't doing well but I felt coherent enough to try and keep my appointments with patients at the hospital. A hallmark of TBI that I now know I had been exhibiting, but hadn't had anyone point out to me at the time, was clouded judgment. Remember that like many others in the medical field, I self-identify as a caregiver and a workaholic, so my primal response to most situations is to push ahead and work. Unfortunately, in the midst of a TBI, it is our more primal functions that win out. Evidence, facts, and logic are missing because that part of the brain, the frontal lobe with executive functioning, just isn't processing. Fortunately, at that time I was dealing primarily with patients suffering carpal tunnel and other low-risk, neuromuscular issues, basic rote memory stuff, so I hadn't unwittingly put anyone in immediate danger. Were my specialty to have been as a cardiologist, hematologist, nephrologist, surgeon, anywhere where intellectual skills and technical ability were potentially life-threatening, I could not have continued to practice. Indeed, I have colleagues in these specialties who had to opt out of practice for up to a year or more due to the effects of "mild" TBI.

Through impaired speech, shaky movements, and dimmed lights I managed to record patient information using a combination of brief statements and directing them to point at the relevant questions and symptoms on the diagnostic sheets. The only person who seemed to clearly know I was struggling was my assistant, Joan. I sensed I was only making life more difficult for those around me. As with many caregivers, when the caregiver themselves need care it can often cause those they regularly care for to become almost angry with them for needing relief from normal, daily responsibilities they'd always handled. This extended to my patients and even some referral doctors who would ultimately find me unavailable. Attempting to carry on, I just barely made it through Tuesday, taking a cab to work and catching a lift home again, but by the Wednesday following the accident the charade was up.

Dr. Kalev Freeman, working with several other researchers as part of the Freeman Trauma Physiology Lab, discovered that mild TBI (mTBI) injuries and successive TBIs run a course wherein the symptoms of the injury peak between the three- and five-day mark.[13] Whereas a severe TBI may induce the maximum symptoms immediately, mTBI and recurring low-level traumas (such as what occur in football linemen on every play as their helmets crash together) will build over the coming hours and days. It is exactly this reason why so many TBIs have previously gone undiagnosed or are diagnosed late.

For our military on the battlefield or athletes on the playing field, this flaw in the system can prove fatal. Imagine being Staff Sgt. Armstrong, being told by a doctor whom you respect and trust that everything about you physically is coming back as normal when they are utilizing some of the most modern, technological diagnostic tools. Likewise, imagine this incorrect initial diagnosis serving as the basis for whether or not you might receive treatment or compensation in the future, after continuing to suffer from various symptoms, such as what has happened to Armstrong repeatedly under VA guidelines. As much as my struggle to function was very real to me I felt like I must be crazy, and that I couldn't possibly be as bad off as I'd felt I was because everything kept coming back "normal." And so it goes that this is why many of us who have suffered from an mTBI quickly return to our own field of profession, battle, or play.

When I returned to the hospital Wednesday morning both my mental and physical shape were in rapid decline. My symptoms had hit their crescendo and I went hysterical trying to evaluate one of my patients. By this time, all speech was halted, and I had to communicate through shaky writing and brief notes. Even my patients were very concerned. I was able to find my friend and colleague Dr. Peters once more, thankfully, as the deep confusion and overstimulation had returned in full force.

After another evaluation, which included another CT scan, Dr. Peters stated, "This may seem hard to believe, but I still can't find anything abnormal on the tests," even though he agreed that something obviously wasn't right.

Another member of the ER staff made a call to Terry to come and pick me up as there was no longer any possibility of me continuing to work that day. I sat in the car crying over what a mess I was and my inability to communicate the seriousness of the situation to her, while she opted to stop by the gas station to top off the tank. Thinking of it now I realize just what a huge, awkward scene it had become, in part because I felt that if everyone else believed I was "normal" then I must be, and I must work—but also in part because my only option for a caregiver, a friend, seemed to be unconcerned with my condition. I mean, why stop for gas when I felt like I was losing my brain? Again, I had always been the strong one, and becoming dependent on another person was not something I wished for in the slightest.

I'd planned for an early Christmas celebration trip to Colorado prior to all of this (which obviously was out of the question at this point), meaning I'd already been scheduled off for the next couple of days. I scratched out a note asking Terry to contact the hospital and let them know I'd be out for the next week. Before it was all said and done, I missed more than two weeks of work. I had not missed two weeks of work, cumulatively, in 18 years.

My isolation began in earnest that Wednesday evening when I began my rotation between my bed and my LaZBoy. My balance had become so bad that I gave myself only sponge baths because I feared I would slip and fall in a shower or possibly slip into unconsciousness in the bathtub and drown. I could barely move, and I sat alone throughout the day in as much darkness as I could claim against the daylight outside. No radio nor television played, as I attempted to keep all stimulation, aural and visual, to an absolute minimum. For more than 10 days I only communicated what I absolutely needed to via pen and paper, mostly just when Terry or another friend would show up in the evenings with a bag of Wendy's for dinner. That became as close to any routine that I had during this time—the polar opposite of my life less than a week earlier.

Just days into this process and I'd gone from successful, well-kempt, well-informed physician to someone who would best be described as appearing disheveled and confused. I find no small amount of irony in this description as research being completed in metropolitan areas in both Canada and the United States has uncovered that anywhere between 50 and 70 percent of the homeless population have suffered at least one TBI—if not multiple TBIs.[14] In fact, TBI is one of the strongest predictors of homelessness, as mentioned earlier in this book in regard to many former NFL players, including Iron Mike, as featured in the *Frontline* episode "League of Denial."

According to the National Coalition for Homeless Veterans (NCHV) about 1.4 million veterans are "at risk of homelessness," noting that on any given night the US Department of Housing and Urban Development (HUD) estimates almost 50,000 veterans are homeless.[15] While there is certainly a complex set of factors that lead to homelessness, including shortages of affordable housing and disparity between the job market and the payment of living wages, one of the causes deemed a significant factor in veteran homelessness is a lack of access to healthcare, in particular access to care for PTSD and TBI and other mental and emotional issues. The NCHV demographics show that 51 percent of homeless veterans suffer from a disability; 50 percent of homeless veterans have a serious mental illness; 70 percent have acquired substance abuse problems. These numbers aren't the whole story though; a key number excluded from these homeless heroes are the 140,000 veterans serving time in the state and federal prison systems. Interestingly, over half of these prison veterans served during wartime and received an honorable discharge, while similar numbers (57 percent) are also serving time for violent offenses. Currently, the VA is making strides to end homelessness in our veterans, but until we attack the root cause, until we get our veterans into cognitive rehabilitation and services to bring back their brains in addition to their mind, spirit, and body, we will not solve the problem, only make it better for a while. Our veterans need to be moved off the streets and into homes where proper diagnosis and treatment can begin, or begin again.

When I review information like what the NCHV provides, I am reminded just how much my position as physician has played a role in getting me from that moment in time, where I struggled with even the desire, much less the ability, to keep communicating and to keep on living; how that could have in any other scenario ended up with me actually homeless instead of just looking as if I were. The advantages my socio-economic position provided me meant an enormous amount to my recovery, and this is part of why I am so passionate about sharing what I've learned. I'm hoping that those who might otherwise not find their way back to the light, those who may feel like they have no voice, will use my voice for their recovery.

General (Ret.) Dennis Laich, in his book *Skin in the Game*,[16] explores in depth how the vast majority of our military force is comprised of young men and women who come from backgrounds of poverty or are working poor immigrants who view military service as a path to citizenship. Against all odds many of our country's top athletes started life in abject poverty, fighting for their day of recognition, their stardom, by working hard at their chosen sport throughout grade school. These phenomena aren't merely taking place in the US either. A recent French study looked at the prevalence of injuries suffered by position in the sport of international rugby and found a somewhat unsurprisingly high number of concussions among nearly every position on the field.[17] The use of the "header" in soccer—a move where a player hits the ball with their head as a way to pass or shoot the ball—has also been researched and found to similarly cause frequent mTBI which ultimately, over time, may lead to the same symptoms as any TBI sufferer develops. Both rugby and soccer are seen internationally as a way out of poverty for millions of young, underprivileged men and women around the world the way football, baseball, and basketball are here in the US. As awareness of TBI and the related diseases such as CTE grows, some athletes are choosing to donate their brains for post-mortem research; US Women's National Team soccer star Brandi Chastain is one of those athletes.

In a 2016 interview with *The New York Times* journalist John Branch, Chastain said, "If there's any information to be gleaned off the study of someone like myself, who has played soccer for 40 years, it feels like my responsibility—but not in a burdensome way. People talk about what the '99 group did for women's soccer. They say, 'Oh, you left a legacy for the next generation.' This would be a more substantial legacy—something that could protect and save some kids … If we can learn something, we should."[18]

During the intervening years between my TBI and the writing of this book, research has shown what I instinctively relied upon during my recovery, that the more defined knowledge and mental stimulation a person has prior to their injury, the more likely they will retain some of those tools directly after their TBI, giving them a foundation—albeit possibly just a very small footing—to begin building on once more. My fate was much better because of my experiences, opportunities, and all the information I had stored away which eventually helped me navigate through the dense fog I was experiencing. For many of our nation's young men and women, who are pulled out of poverty by joining military service or pursuing athletics, they may not have had access to the same sorts of experiences, opportunities, and information, not to mention financial resources to find alternate health care and rehabilitation services once injured. This is particularly true of the military member who is discharged to the civilian world without a plan or without assistance to navigate the Veterans Administration health care service. Considering the fact that nearly half of our military members reside in rural communities, the access to care and information becomes an even greater struggle.

My status as a physician meant that those consultants and staff members interacting with me knew I was different because they knew the person I had been just the day before at work. They understood what family members and others seemed unwilling to acknowledge, that it wasn't that I was crazy, or on drugs; they believed me when I asked for help—even if they struggled to find the problem—and the fact that they believed me was the number-one key. As previously discussed, often a TBI patient is mistaken for a drug user, and in many cases (that we'll learn more about later in the text), those who suffer TBI and don't know how to get help will turn to alcohol or other controlled substances to attempt to self-medicate, and once they finally do end up in an ER the attempted self-medication further masks the TBI at the root of the problem.

My fortune wasn't just in being under the care of my colleagues either. I had insurance and other financial resources that allowed for me to follow as many diagnostic and treatment paths as I cared to, and the sort of take-charge personality that I think lends itself to recovery—to the constant self-directed sort of exercises required to rehabilitate the brain, not unlike what is required to rehabilitate a torn muscle.

What very few young military families have are the financial resources to buy their way through a difficult and in many ways broken health care system. A quick search of crowdfunding websites such as You Caring returns an endless list of veterans and their families requesting support for issues associated with TBI and PTSD, such as a number of campaigns to tackle homelessness, TBI research, and individual or project funding of programs to deal with the symptoms of PTSD. With a lack of specific protocols for diagnosis and treatment, the cost of trial and error treatment can be staggering. Our young returning veterans should have access to care through the VA system, but that system is in turmoil and is unprepared to diagnose, much less treat, TBI in the majority of the centers. Even the symptoms associated with PTSD, often a follow-on disability to TBI, are difficult to get treatment for through the current VA system. Yet, a traumatic brain injury diagnosis should be made as soon as possible after the injury, with immediate treatment in order to achieve the best results.

Suicide amongst TBI sufferers is eight times more common than amongst the general public. Suicide among our returning service members and veterans in the US has been called an "epidemic" by many, including some of our enlightened leaders on Capitol Hill. By 2012 the number of service members dying in battle, even with the ongoing operations in Afghanistan, was lower than the number of suicides committed by veterans back home. According to reporting by NPR, 349 veterans committed suicide in 2012 while 295 soldiers died in combat that year.[19] This is not just symptomatic of our returning heroes either. Several suicides linked to TBI, and specifically CTE, in football players and other athletes are beginning to surface as well. To date 90 former NFL players have been diagnosed post-mortem with CTE; several have died by suicide. In February 2016 extreme sport star BMX bike rider Dave Mirra died of a self-inflicted gunshot wound. Results of brain tests carried out by neuropathologist Lili-Naz Hazrati, PhD, MD, FRCPC, of the University of Toronto and the Canadian Concussion Centre, found the athlete had the progressive disease chronic traumatic encephalopathy, or CTE.[20] This was the disease process described in the book *Concussion*,[21] which dealt with the life of Dr. Bennet Omalu, played in the subsequent movie by Will Smith.[22] Omalu defined the pathology which accompanies years of brain injury.

Staff Sgt. Armstrong said that he was given several prescriptions by VA doctors in an attempt to treat his symptoms, even though this ultimately seemed to mask his actual problems of thinking and processing. "In the middle of the worst veteran and soldier suicide rates we've seen, the VA is handing out these anti-depressants and other sorts of drugs which have side effects like causing suicidal thoughts," Armstrong said.

In my interview with him, retired Army Sgt. Wendell Guillermo said he'd had a similar experience.

"When I went to the VA they had me do a battery of tests and then they gave me this whole concoction of medication and, at least for me, it didn't do me well—it made things worse—I had no feelings or emotions at all, nothing," Guillermo said.

Similarly, standout running back Jonathan Wells said that, "anything you've got an injury for, the NFL has a pill for you."

"When the pain is bearable I try not to use any pain medications because I've been there and done that," he said when asked about opioid addiction. "Tylenol #3, Vicodin, all sorts of pills. These pills they give you to take so you can play keep you high all day so once you're off the field you really can't function and you're basically just self-medicating."

Even for people who have an injury such as a broken bone, one that doesn't tax their mental capacity at all, a visit to any ER in the US can be very stressful and taxing. At this point I feel as though it goes without saying, but when your brain is so fogged in that you can't even deal with having the lights on, dealing with the stress and frustration associated with navigating multiple forms, and long periods of waiting for responses, for appointments, for answers, in and of itself is too much for many TBI sufferers who are experiencing confusion and all other manners of difficulties.

The one resource I was lacking in up front that had put me at a disadvantage, and is also an issue shared with so many of our veterans suffering a TBI, is going into care without an advocate. For TBI sufferers who don't have any family, or whose partners can't afford to take time off to provide advocacy and further care, those TBI sufferers are at the mercy of what the staff on duty know, or do not know, about TBI. If my advocacy could impact just one thing in regard to our system of care, it would be to guarantee an advocate who is truly working only for the TBI patient's best interests. We must assist the caregivers for our TBI patients; the course is arduous at best and impossible at worst—the system does not work when it requires a patient to self-report because often their brain is so scrambled that they just can't.

I can't stress enough how important a positive, proactive advocate can be, not just for the purpose of recovering from a TBI, but for even just the sake of keeping the injured alive. This isn't just about situations like mine, where there was concern as to whether or not I'd wake up from my sleep—where I should have had someone willing to follow along with the prescribed treatment plan which included waking me up hourly, to check that

I was still alive and not comatose. This is about the all-too-familiar drug overdosing we hear about regularly on the news from people who attempt to self-medicate their problems away. This is about the suicidal thoughts that become all too real for TBI sufferers who don't see another path, who feel like too much of a burden to be worth saving.

Distinguished Professor of Psychology at Florida State University Dr. Thomas Joiner, working with his research team in the Joiner Lab, developed the theory of suicide attempt and execution which requires the connecting of three crucial components, two of which are virtually built into every TBI patient's care plan, or lack of care plan, as it often is.

In his book and lectures titled *Why People Die by Suicide*,[23] Joiner advances his theory that feelings of perceived burdensomeness and also of thwarted belongingness, when combined with the physical and mental capability for suicide, will likely result in death by suicide.

Without anyone to actively take charge and advocate for me, and to provide care for me even if I was uncomfortable about giving up my role as the caregiver, I found my feeling of burdensomeness growing exponentially with each passing day. This feeling was the number-one factor contributing to my personal desire to die (possibly by committing suicide), and I struggle with even discussing it here because I desperately don't want anyone to consider death or suicide as a viable option.

Considering the numbers we've discussed previously that were related to self-medication rates of our returning veterans, the recorded number of suicides versus accidental drug overdose, becomes much grayer than strict black and white. Unfortunately, as a physician, I had, at least conceptually, multiple potential sources for controlled substances that might either act as medication or as a suicidal prescription.

Fortunately for me, I was incapable of overcoming my fear of death. I couldn't think of any way of killing myself that I was mentally prepared to carry out, let alone physically. I could barely use a telephone at this point, so how was I supposed to manage a firearm and efficiently end my life? I have an aversion to pain, so many of the more basic options were also off the table. Ultimately what moved my thoughts out of this darkness was realizing I did not want to burden my family with the knowledge that I'd committed suicide.

The lack of any solid TBI protocol or even firm understanding of how the injury interacts with the symptoms automatically creates a feeling of being outside the system, of no longer belonging. Searching, often fruitlessly, for answers, especially if you're doing so mostly on your own as I was, only perpetuates both the feeling of being alone as well as the feeling of burdening others—clinicians as well as friends and family. I remember thinking at times how I was wasting my time and other people's time because I found myself at dead ends time and again.

Joiner, in a lecture at the Sidney J. Blatt memorial series hosted by Ben Gurion University, explained that it is fearlessness that ultimately moves an individual from being potentially suicidal to executing a serious, often successful, attempt at suicide.[24] Drugs are also known to significantly lower inhibitions while heightening negative thought patterns by tapping into more primal thought processes, adding the high rate of self-medicating sufferers to the higher risk levels.

"You can see it in their eyes, their blink rate is significantly slower," Joiner said in the lecture. "They're focused and ready to do something. When you're about to perform as a concert pianist. When you're about to go into the boxing ring. When you're about to commit suicide.

"You have to be focused when you stare down the deep seeded fear of death we're all born with in order to kill oneself. There are a lot of people who very much want to die, but at the very last moment they blink, they don't do it. It's the ones that don't blink that we lose."

Football player Wells said that like many of his fellow athletes he's stared down suicide as well, something he's sadly known most of his life, and is ironically inextricable from his passion for football.

His brother, Kenneth Wells Jr., committed suicide at 12 years old in the family home. Football and athletics in general became a way for Jonathan to keep busy and move past this tragedy. After sustaining repeated trauma to his head while playing in the National Football League, Jonathan himself had once again come to know the act and ideation of suicide.

"I talk to a lot of former athletes I played with who have the same problems I suffer from: headaches, depression, pain, memory loss," Wells said. "I've had a few friends and players who I looked up to commit suicide this past year. A while back I contemplated driving off a bridge while driving home to New Orleans after visiting my doctor, Kelly Ryder, in Baton Rouge. I was crying uncontrollably and stopped on the bridge. I called my fiancé and thank GOD she answered because she talked me down and all the way to my parents' home. If she hadn't answered I'm not sure I'd still be here. I was in a bad place. I ended up checking into a hospital that night. When I returned to Ohio, I started to see a psychiatrist, and continue to do so."

Current research suggests between 20-40 percent of TBI patients will engage in some form of substance abuse within the first year after the injury.[25] This often plays out in one of three ways: using alcohol, marijuana, or opiates to slow brain processes even further than the injury itself has slowed them; or using caffeine, nicotine, amphetamines, or cocaine to speed brain processing up; or attempting to get outside of the brain by using psychotropic medicines, LSD, and others.

This chapter opened by explaining that dark is dark, and every TBI sufferer knows this. Unfortunately, the darkness we began this chapter with is all too often merely the beginning of the spiral we've been exploring and one I personally slid much of the way down. Without proper protocols and without a one-on-one support mechanism, the typical scenario runs from injury, to self-medicating *cum* substance abuse, to unemployment, homelessness, and eventually incarceration or suicide. So typical is this spiral that Dr. Peter Breggin, noted psychiatrist, was asked to testify before the Veterans Affairs Committee of the US House of Representatives on the topic "Exploring the Relationship between Medication and Veteran Suicide[26]" and to ultimately work in partnership with the Veterans Defense Project in 2014 to develop an "Attorney's Guide to Defending Veterans in Criminal Court."[27]

In both cases, Breggin states that, "Patients with head injury are especially susceptible to the adverse effects of all psychoactive substances ... [and that] ... the symptoms of TBI and PTSD can be difficult to distinguish from each other, and frequently aggravate each other ... [yet there are]... No [psychiatric] medications approved for the treatment of TBI or closed head injury in general, but psychiatric drugs are nonetheless commonly given to patients with TBI (and) to patients with PTSD. As a result, patients with PTSD, TBI, or both are routinely given psychiatric drugs, often many at one time."

Breggin's conclusions drawn from US Food and Drug Administration documentation correlate that young adults through the age of 24 who used psychoactive substances, especially prescribed antidepressants, showed an increased rate of suicidality and violence. He writes, "If TBI and or PTSD remain inadequately treated over a period of months and years, both are likely to cause similar clinical symptoms of cognitive impairment, apathy or indifference, social withdrawal, fatigue, depression and suicidality, emotional instability or lability, and a general limitation on the quality of life."

TBI and PTSD frequently coexist, the former representing a physical injury to the brain cells, the latter an abnormal chemical injury.

Brigadier General (Ret.) Gerald D. Griffin, MD, PharmD, further explained the brain chemical imbalance following an mTBI which is associated with PTSD. This change in chemical structure occurs as the brain tries to normalize function that has been interrupted by stress and trauma, and often leads to a decreased ability for the body to even fight off infection. That is, the chemical insult to the brain following trauma not only results in a lack of psychological well-being, but a lack of physical well-being, as well, with increased risk of infection and further health compromise. In other words, in the struggle for the brain to return to normal, the body's well-being is threatened.[28]

Dark is dark, but once we've entered this downward spiral it would seem as if it can always get ever darker.

CHAPTER FOUR

FLICKER OF LIGHT

Intelligence did not get me out of this—for as much as I had accomplished in my life academically and intellectually prior to the TBI, the wiping clear of my brain was a very steep drop for me to fall, and served only to make me that much more depressed about my situation. Likewise an athlete or soldier who has relied so heavily upon their mental and physical capabilities can be devastated by losing that edge due to imbalance or loss of motor functionality; taking away the one thing that has always served a person well in life is taking away perceived self-worth. One important factor regarding TBI recovery is that the sufferer can't just change their mind and decide to be OK, or to think positively, or really to control their thoughts at all. This type of injury can rob a person of not just physical controls but of even the ability to rationalize between accurate and deceptive thoughts.

Caregivers to TBI patients can play the role of helping the sufferer to receive positive reinforcement, and this is no small task. Frontal lobe damage, in particular, can remove all filters for both speech and reaction, meaning that TBI sufferers are more likely to lash out both verbally and physically in response to agitation.

In extreme cases of severe TBI, not the focus of this book, the situation can even escalate into injurious or fatal scenarios for the caregiver. Dr. Neil Brooks at the University of Glasgow found that over a five-year study of 42 individuals with severe TBI, threats of violence increased 15 percent in one year after sustaining their head injury, and climbed to 54 percent five years after. Ultimately at the five-year follow-up consultation, 20 percent had been reported for assaulting their relatives at least once and 31 percent of the patients had faced legal problems.[29]

In the cases of mTBI that we are focused on here, violence directed toward others is less frequent as more of the frontal lobe connections still exist. Although, as discussed previously, self-harm through substance abuse or suicide attempt is common and may become injurious to caregivers without any intention on behalf of the TBI patient.

Fortunately, I fell into the mTBI group and have never been a violent person; and as much as I may have wanted to unleash a verbal tirade on those who still thought I was faking, I was still incapable of speaking. Throughout this time, I had few people checking in on me—few friends and no family believing that I could be that impaired as to not take care of myself.

I remember my assistant, Joan, coming over to the house before going to the office. This was on a Friday, about two weeks after the accident. My friend, Terry, was at work when Joan arrived early in the morning. Joan immediately became concerned that I was still unable to speak coherently, and that my symptoms such as lethargy and fatigue had only become worse since she'd last seen me at work. Using pen and paper I was able to communicate with her that I needed her to contact a colleague and former teacher of mine whom I knew would be able to help.

During my medical training I had studied under a brilliant physician who was very skilled in TBI specialty care. Joan assisted me with calling him and consulting with him over the phone concerning what had happened to me and how my symptoms were not improving. I did my best to convey what I could to Joan via pen and paper, so that she could communicate with him, and I held on to my hope. I knew that he would understand, just as Joan and Dr. Peters had, that I was in crisis.

Of the myriad of issues related to the state of health care in the United States today, one of the more pressing issues is how the economic dynamic has impacted a doctor's curiosity. What I mean is that historically (I believe) one thing that separates good physicians from excellent clinicians and healers is an inherent curiosity about human physiology, biology, chemistry, and the role that mind, body, and spirit are playing out in the disease process; in other words, the desire to solve puzzles. The ability to see the future—what will work and what will fail—is what makes a great physician. Equally as important is the commitment of the time necessary to solve the puzzle, a true necessity for traumatic brain injury care. Today, however, more and more doctors are tied to protocols set up by the health care industry, which prioritizes payment by productive minute—or as it is otherwise referred to in some circles, the Relative Value Units (RVU).

In a publicly available online document authored by Merritt Hawkins, an AMN Healthcare Company, titled "RVU Based Physician Compensation and Productivity -Ten Recommendations for Determining Physician Compensation/Productivity Through Relative Value Units," the company states that "volume-based metrics attached to the number of patients physicians see" is a prominent method for calculating revenue.[30] As part of their list of 10 recommendations, only one of them, number six on the list, addresses quality of care—and in doing so states that Merritt Hawkins recommends offering a "quality incentive"—which they suggest will allow doctors to worry less about revenue generation. Quantifying payment based on the number of patients a doctor can pass through the door each day, as opposed to the quality of care the patients receive, removes not only the incentive for a doctor to let their inquisitive mind wander, but actively punishes them financially for it.

This is why TBI patients will only begin to receive the care they deserve when we train enough physicians and research doctors willing to sit at the table and play chess, as I see it. Every move a doctor makes, whether it be prescribing drugs or setting up a team approach of therapists and other specialists, can elicit a response that may or may not be positive for the TBI sufferer. The injured brain can play dirty sometimes, and if a doctor is unwilling or unable to spend the time weighing every move and looking at the potential outcomes, he or she just might get rooked.

For this very reason I believed reaching out to a teaching hospital was my best bet at survival. I knew physicians there were up to the challenge, and due to the large number of patients, my colleagues had dealt with this hundreds of times before. My colleague requested that Joan put me on the phone, and ever so methodically and caringly, took my history by having me answer in a series of grunts—one grunt, YES; two grunts, NO. By the end of the call, he assured me that he understood my current condition and offered to phone in a prescription for me of amantadine, a drug often used to help treat Parkinson's disease and conditions similar to Parkinson's. While research about the impact of amantadine on TBI recovery is still very inconclusive, a placebo-controlled study completed in 2012, conducted across 11 clinical sites in three countries, found that rates of recovery appeared to be about two weeks faster for patients receiving the drug versus those receiving the placebo.[31] As with most drug interactions with brain functions, there is still a wide gap between what is known about why these drugs work for some people and not for others, or exactly what reaction they cause that creates a positive (or negative) response. Primarily amantadine is known to cause nerve arousal, promoting the release of dopamine and blocking re-uptake post-synaptically. In more layman terms, the belief is that amantadine causes the disconnected nerve synapses to begin communicating again through the release of dopamine. Specifically, according to the study, "the rate of recovery was more rapid in the amantadine group, affecting functionally meaningful behaviors such as consistent responses to commands, intelligible speech, reliable yes-or-no communication, and functional-object use."

Before leaving my house around 10 a.m., Joan let my friend Terry know that I had a prescription waiting for me at the pharmacy, and Terry agreed to pick it up and bring it to me. Joan had offered to get it for me, but I sent her on to the office, knowing that it would take a couple hours to fill the prescription. I had no idea that Terry, who worked nearby, would wait until the end of the day to pick it up and bring it to me around 8 p.m. that night.

Apparently, my friend never thought that I may have needed it or wanted it sooner, even though this was the first specific attempt to use medication to potentially help my recovery. I sat there waiting for Terry in silence, in the dark, for ten hours for what I hoped would be my "miracle cure." When Terry finally arrived I was hysterical, making a mostly unintelligible screaming noise at my friend, like the bark of a fox. I know I had little right to be so demanding, but I was desperate for a "fix," anything that would help jump start my then totally sluggish brain. I felt that even though Terry was not a family member nor close friend, there would be at least some understanding of my desperation. I understand, now, that looking through my lens of a confused, agitated TBI survivor, this may have been a tad irrational. Nevertheless, I respond very quickly to patients in this same situation because I understand that definitely, time is relative when your brain is in slow motion.

I scratched out on paper, "I would NEVER have kept you waiting for your medicine," which was met with pure surprise, before I ripped open the bottle, as if I were an addict looking for a fix—and in a way I was looking for a fix, a brain fix. Although I had no recollection at the time what amantadine was or did, I trusted my colleague at the hospital and knew he would find a way to fix me.

As I waited patiently in my LaZBoy, one hour passed, and then another. I began losing hope that this drug might do anything more for my brain than the Wendy's hamburger I'd had for dinner. Delicious as it was, it did not prove to be brain food. Around 10 p.m. I began to get up to go to bed when I became hyper-aware of some sort of electricity in my body, that same sort of feeling you get when your hair begins to stand on end. Something was about to happen and my first reaction was to think that I was about to have a seizure, a recurrent theme in my recovery, as it turned out. I considered my options and decided that if I was going to seize, letting it happen while I sat in the padded lazy chair was my safest bet. Ten minutes into feeling like this I noticed my vision clearing—not clearing gradually, as if you were focusing a lens on a camera, but clearing rapidly, in a series of distinct views, like the click of an automatic camera as the vision improved in clarity and dimension. Click, click, and five clicks later, I no longer saw double vision, and my world became sharp and clear.

I could see! I mean I could really see!

For the past two weeks I'd suffered from fuzzy vision, everything caked in a hazy gauze effect and doubled—the effect irritating my senses and serving as a constant visual reminder of my disabled state. Now though, like a switch had flipped, my vision had sharpened. I was struck dumb with joy over this new development. I remained sitting in silence, until, at about 11:30 p.m., I spoke. I didn't just utter a few garbled syllables nor just a single yes/no type word like I'd been able to use off and on over the past couple of weeks, but an actual, complete, full, and intelligible sentence—one that I will never forget.

"Why didn't you get this for me sooner?!" I said slowly, yet clearly, to Terry, and Terry understood my inquiry, and that was my flicker of hope.

I honestly am not trying to be too critical of my non-medically trained friend. Although we had been friends for a couple years, we were not that close, and pretty much led separate lives that came together rather loosely due in a large margin to my independent nature. I prided myself that I did not rely on anyone; the fact that I now needed to rely on so many people was very hard for me to accept. Terry had no medical training, and I looked as strong as I had before the injury. My friend was not accustomed, however, to looking into the eyes of a person who has suffered brain trauma. Even a seemingly insignificant blow to the brain can cause disruption—can cause the eyes of the person to dull. It is as if they are focusing on an object 1,000 feet away. We use phrases like "zombie" and "blank stare," or, more frequently, "lights out; nobody home." Once you have looked into the eyes of someone with a TBI, you do not forget that stare. I became quite familiar with it—from looking into a mirror for over four months.

There it was. I knew that amantadine had hit the light switch. I could see, and I could speak, and it happened all of a sudden. I stayed awake until after midnight, hoping for additional points of light, of recovery, but none came. That being what it was, I was ecstatic over what I'd regained, and I don't mean my voice and my vision, I mean the glimmer of hope that had become so much diminished.

In the morning I awoke in my pre-amantadine condition. I was crestfallen that the recovery hadn't been permanent. My vision, though clearer than it was previously, was not sharp, and I could not speak, again. I took my next dose of amantadine and after another short interlude once again regained my sight and speech. Over time I came to realize that the half-life of my dosage was about six hours. That first day I'd gone about 12 hours between doses and over the coming several months as I was continuing to take amantadine I never let myself go that long between doses. Instead, I set alarms for every six hours, round the clock, so that I wouldn't miss a dose. I took amantadine like I was hooked on it because it was the only thing I knew that linked my former self to my current self, and I desperately wanted my former self back.

What we didn't have an understanding of at the time, but is becoming more and more accepted as research continues to move forward on TBI treatment, is that the brain functions much like any individual nerve cell; it is an all-or-nothing machine. I didn't have a series of small steps to getting each function back, I didn't see a little bit better each day, or speak a little bit more clearly each day; no, I spoke unintelligibly and then spoke clearly, I had blurry double vision and then had clear vision. You don't crawl, then stagger, then walk when recovering from a TBI. Instead the neural pathway is laid down, and when the final connection is made, you are all better.

This is not to confuse anyone that "all better" means the same as before the injury; that isn't accurate either. To be clear, becoming all better means that the full functionality had returned, but what I did with that functionality in some cases needed to be re-taught, and when you are relearning things you don't always relearn them as well as you had originally. Regardless, this is all new intelligence being discovered in TBI care, and there is so much more left to discover. I also find it important to bear in mind that I was only a couple of weeks into this process, and only because of my prior connections to the medical field did this potential recovery option present itself so early on. Most of our veterans have been suffering the effects of TBI for years, often without either diagnosis or rehab. Worse still is the number of them who have opted to either self-medicate, or who have been put on a rotating cocktail of psychotropic prescription drugs, or both.

Matt Gossard is an 82nd Airborne Paratrooper who suffered a TBI playing in a high school basketball game, an injury that led to hospitalization. He then went on to survive three IED explosions during a seven-month tour of duty in Iraq. On a training parachute jump at Ft. Bragg, he suffered a loss-of-consciousness injury, again. Gossard had been the picture of health and fitness. However, as part of a recovery process he had been prescribed oxycodone, a pain medicine several times more addictive than heroin. This medication, which is often in the news, was originally formulated only for terminal patients. Who knows whether or not a TBI actually may increase the possibility of addiction to oxycodone, as it does to so many other substances such as alcohol and even caffeine.

After battling an addiction to oxycodone for over a year at Ft. Bragg, he was discharged from military service and left to his own devices to deal with what eventually turned into a multifaceted problem of substance abuse that he battled with for a couple years, before overcoming this physician-imposed addiction. Gossard's recovery program included cognitive retraining—re-booting the brain—and he worked very hard toward his recovery. He now works alongside the Ohio attorney general's task force for opiate addiction, as director of the Champions Network, and is assisting his military brothers and sisters, as well as his community, in overcoming the addiction. In addition, he is completing his college degree and is a testimony to how hard you must work through a TBI and the co-morbidities associated with being "out of your brain." I honestly don't know how anyone in this position survives, and I am motivated to make sure that in the future our heroes and their families aren't left to battle undiagnosed injuries alone.

Amantadine was working for me and I was very grateful, but like the multiple medications being handed out to other TBI sufferers, it isn't a silver bullet; it doesn't work for everyone. The key to using medication to stimulate recovery and battle the symptoms during the intervening time between injury and recovery is two-fold. First, as is practiced by the Ohio State University (OSU) TBI clinic, is to make small, incremental shifts in medication. Secondly, as mentioned above, most people who suffer a TBI, particularly our returning veterans, have lingered for years using medicines that only at best deal with symptoms, or they self-medicate, which often leads to the demise of relationships, legal issues, and homelessness. In fact, following the end of the Vietnam War, those veterans suffering various ailments averaged about 15 years between leaving service and encountering homelessness. For the veterans of Operation Iraqi Freedom (OIF) and Operation Enduring Freedom (OEF) (Afghanistan) this timeline had decreased exponentially, down to only 15 weeks. Part of what studies are suggesting will make an impact on both prevention of the co-morbidity issues of drug abuse and homelessness, as well as improve actual rehabilitation and recovery from TBI and the associated PTSD, is greatly increasing the number of touch points clinicians have with their TBI (and especially mTBI) patients.

Diagnosed initially with PTSD, Sgt. Guillermo received a TBI after a grenade went off in the middle of his compromised overwatch position during the first elections held in Iraq following the Saddam Hussein regime.

"It was seven of us total including our platoon leader and our radio operator," Guillermo explained to me in an interview. "I'd had my back turned and was taking a knee to pack my ruck because we were about to head out when I heard someone yell—GRENADE! After the explosion I used my training to help save one buddy's life while we awaited medivac to the Mosul hospital. It was a surreal experience, felt like time just kind of slowed down as the grenade went off. Initially it felt like a flash concussion and not a big deal.

"I was fortunate not to be one of the guys sent back into battle immediately. Then, mainly after I separated [from military service], I noticed more and more that I had moments where bright light was giving me headaches and stuff like that. Then, it was until about two years after separation that I was fully diagnosed with TBI and PTSD," Guillermo said. "If I had any advice for other soldiers it would be to get help immediately and not to fall for the stigma around a PTSD or TBI diagnosis because the faster you get help the more likely you'll recover. In the end, that's for your well-being."

Current standards average the time between appointments being about four to six weeks. Knowing now how rapidly changes can take place in the brain, physicians following patients with TBI are advocating for weekly consultations at first, eventually moving to a bi-weekly schedule as recovery proceeds. This is crucial in regard to treating the root cause, the TBI itself, as opposed to focusing on symptom management. This is much the same as a 12-step program that may be beneficial in the short term for keeping sobriety, but without identifying and relieving the root cause of the self-medication and addiction, sobriety is mostly for naught. Likewise, finding subsidized housing for homeless veterans is a necessary task in the effort to bring them back into the mainstream; but ultimately without addressing the cause of their emotional issues, steady employment and housing aren't sustainable. I can't advocate for anything that promotes a rebound type behavior, which is why it is so important to begin serious diagnosis and treatment of TBI as quickly as possible and with as few delays as possible.

Thankfully, TBI is finally being considered a chronic illness, and not just an injury to be fixed and forgotten. Care facilities—even those in the VA system—are beginning to accept that post-rehabilitation sufferers of a TBI are still likely to have recurring bouts of depression, headaches, and epilepsy. They may also develop Parkinson's or Alzheimer's disease later in life, and now, thanks to the work of Ann McKee, MD, neuropathologist at Boston University and Director of the Neuropathology Service for the New England Veterans Administration Medical Centers, we know that chronic traumatic encephalopathy, CTE, is also a possibility.[32]

The flicker of light that I found for myself required taking the risk of reaching out for help, and allowing myself to trust the judgment of others such as Joan and the TBI clinic. This is similar to the flicker of light we're seeing in TBI research more broadly as well. As recently as March 2016, the NFL finally admitted to the link between football and CTE, no longer suggesting that players had merely had their "bell rung" in play, but that their violent sport had in fact created repetitious TBI conditions.[33]

Neuroscience researcher Amanda Marie Cardinale reminds us though, in her article for *PsychCentral*, that although the headlines about TBI are increasing exponentially, the actual treatments have yet to change significantly.[34] "One out of three military service members are returning home with a traumatic brain injury in addition to other mental health issues such as PTSD," Cardinale wrote. "Three years of data collected from 10 US brain injury rehabilitation facilities shows that there is a focus on physical, speech, and occupational therapy, but psychological well-being seems to be greatly overlooked."

As Jonathan Wells put it regarding the legal settlement he and several thousand other ex-NFL players are seeking against the NFL for their TBI-related treatments, "The suicide rate is important. That transition out of sports was a really dark time for me, for a lot of us. I spent 20 years playing football and when I left I had to basically start over from scratch. I can imagine it's the same for soldiers."

"There's not a lot out there in terms of support once you leave the NFL. They only provide you five more years of health insurance, and you won't be able to prove a diagnosis like Parkinson's until much later, and they can't even diagnose CTE until you're dead," Wells said. "But still this is a tough one. Football was such a good sport for me. We all made a choice to play but obviously there was a lot of information withheld from us too. So I wouldn't discourage a kid but I would say they need to be very honest with themselves and the coach. If you see stars or black spots do whatever you need to take care of yourself first."

The flicker of light is there, but if we don't advocate daily we may quickly find the spotlight of the press and any increased research on TBI fading back into the darkness.

CHAPTER FIVE

LOOKING FOR THE LIGHTHOUSE

When I was four years old, my grandfather gave me a gift I cherish to this day: the poem "Desiderata" by Max Ehrmann, scripted in a gothic font across a small ceramic piece that I now keep on my kitchen counter as a sort of mantra. It's important enough to my life that I want to share it here.

"Desiderata"

Go placidly amid the noise and haste,
and remember what peace there may be in silence.
As far as possible without surrender
be on good terms with all persons.
Speak your truth quietly and clearly;
and listen to others,
even the dull and the ignorant;
they too have their story.

Avoid loud and aggressive persons,

they are vexations to the spirit.

If you compare yourself with others,

you may become vain and bitter;

for always there will be greater and lesser persons than yourself.

Enjoy your achievements as well as your plans.

Keep interested in your own career, however humble;

it is a real possession in the changing fortunes of time.

Exercise caution in your business affairs;

for the world is full of trickery.

But let this not blind you to what virtue there is;

many persons strive for high ideals;

and everywhere life is full of heroism.

Be yourself.

Especially, do not feign affection.

Neither be cynical about love;

for in the face of all aridity and disenchantment

it is as perennial as the grass.

Take kindly the counsel of the years,

gracefully surrendering the things of youth.

Nurture strength of spirit to shield you in sudden misfortune.

But do not distress yourself with dark imaginings.

Many fears are born of fatigue and loneliness.

Beyond a wholesome discipline,

be gentle with yourself.

You are a child of the universe,

no less than the trees and the stars;

you have a right to be here.

And whether or not it is clear to you,
no doubt the universe is unfolding as it should.
Therefore be at peace with God,
whatever you conceive Him to be,
and whatever your labors and aspirations,
in the noisy confusion of life keep peace with your soul.
With all its sham, drudgery, and broken dreams,
it is still a beautiful world.
Be cheerful.
Strive to be happy. – *Max Ehrmann 1927*

While several of the phrases found within this poem speak deeply to me, I believe that it is this last section, beginning with "Therefore be at peace with God, whatever you conceive Him to be," that requires closer consideration in regard to our topic. You must believe in something to come back from an injury like a TBI—faith in God, faith in science, in yourself, in your family—if you don't find the faith to believe recovery is possible then I believe you won't find the motivation to work as hard as is necessary to recover.

This sentiment is difficult to comprehend for many caregivers and outsiders to the TBI experience. When you consider the rigor and effort required to make it through training camp, boot camp, or through a war zone it becomes extremely difficult to imagine not having the fortitude to simply overcome a TBI on one's own. For many of our military, though, this is the reality. Going into battle depends on how your training has prepared you to accept the challenge. With a TBI though, even our medical providers don't have a solid training plan. There is no boot camp for tackling

TBI, and stepping into the darkness alone can be very difficult if not life changing for too many, and life ending for a few. Brain injury takes away all preparedness for even simple everyday tasks.

For me, calling upon God's grace, that is, the power in my world, is transformative, so why wouldn't I let my body and spirit participate in bringing back my brain? My own belief in a Divine Being and Divine Providence doesn't discount anyone else's (non) belief, because this energy that connects us all is what is important regardless of how you conceive of it, and tapping into that power is what will help us survive those darkest of moments. For many others, and sometimes for myself, it is the serenity prayer that really crystallizes what must be done:

God grant me the serenity to accept the things I cannot change, courage to change the things I can, and the wisdom to know the difference.

Replace that word *God* however you need to so that you can make sense of this and find the serenity, courage, and wisdom necessary to survive the TBI recovery process.

At this point in my story I'm a few weeks into my TBI recovery and my lighthouse in the storm that kept me focused was the medical science which had brought me amantadine. I put my faith in the fact that if my physician was able to bring me the recovery I'd found simply through this medicine, there would be other treatments to be discovered too, and the efforts of these research doctors would not be lost on me.

Therapist Remy Hilchey, MA, CCC-SLP, who has been working with the Veteran's Administration Hospital of Fresno, California developing a therapy program specifically targeted at combat veterans suffering TBI and PTSD is one such individual. In 2011, Hilchey and her colleague Frances Pomaville, PhD, CCC-SLP, introduced a model for an Academic Prep Group in order to assist these veterans to return to school after leaving the military.[35] Ultimately this therapy was introducing what we'll call the serenity prayer strategy, or the acceptance-courage-wisdom strategy for the non-believers in the audience. This strategy is not completely removed from the 12-step program traditions of Alcoholics Anonymous and other addiction-related services. As I've mentioned before, this is good for bringing about some relief, and hopefully during that period of relief allowing some space and physical and mental capacity to overcome the root issues of the TBI.

First comes acceptance of the current state of being: some level of cognitive disability and a goal of recovery, knowing that it can't be done alone.

Second is finding the courage to work towards recovery. This step will include others, such as how Hilchey and Pomaville embraced a group setting to bring together veterans with TBI and PTSD to bolster each other's efforts and learn from one another. Courage and faith are closely coupled as Ancient Roman Senator Marcus Tullius Cicero famously observed, "A man of courage is also full of faith"—for faith is the belief something can be done, while courage is making it happen. Not unlike when entering a dark and unfamiliar room, having the faith that you'll be safe in that space is what allows you the courage to step into it—and when there's someone else by your side, it multiplies the effect.

Third in this model is finding the wisdom to understand that things will never be exactly the same as they were prior to the injury. Knowing what is recoverable as opposed to what will require new strategies is critical to moving forward with your life. As a personal example, I will never be the left-brained person I once was, and at the time this bothered me a lot. My numbers sense was off and I kept writing the wrong dates down—for someone once so devoted to math and statistics I was finding even simple arithmetic difficult. At first I brushed it off, thinking that at any moment it would all return, but by four weeks I was not improving as I had hoped. Ultimately I discovered that by engaging more with the creativity centers found in my right brain I could still find intellectual stimulation and new ways forward in my mission to bring light to the TBI epidemic.

Hilchey is a natural-born healer, and she knows about TBI rehabilitation intimately because her husband, Jarid, is a combat veteran recovering from both a TBI and PTSD. In an interview, Hilchey explained how her programs work and some of the impacts they have had.

"There are always a variety of abilities affected because people with PTSD and TBI have different sets of strengths and weaknesses, both before the injury and after, but overall the general issues are: attention deficits, memory issues, nightmares, pain, sadness, guilt, and frustration. Often the people around them don't understand because everything looks normal from the outside," Hilchey said. "Although you can't see it, their brains are functioning in very different ways than before. It can be very particular from patient to patient as to how much they can accept and work through at a given time."

According to Hilchey, the key up front is to provide as much education to both the TBI sufferer and their caregivers as possible and to establish a rapport with them, so that she can understand where the most critical needs are.

"I like to speak with the families to see where they're coming from and then adjust my treatment plans. They're going through so much and it takes a variety of outlets and interventions for some people to respond. Over time I've found myself acting as a mother, a cheerleader, a sounding board, or even as a drill sergeant. I will have a 'come-to-Jesus' moment if someone is having a pity-party for too long, because while we have to find honor and acceptance of where we are when we start the recovery process, we have to move it forward as well," Hilchey said.

Most of Hilchey's work on combat veteran rehab (outside of that with her husband at home), had been at the VA hospital in Fresno. During the modeling period for the Academic Prep Group, Hilchey and Pomaville determined that the prevalence of TBI and PTSD in combat veterans ranged from 10 to 15 percent between the years 2005-2012. According to reporting from the Defense and Veterans Brain Injury Center (DVBIC), the total numbers for all military TBI from the year 2000-2015 is 344,030[36]. In the DVBIC report, the DoD claims: "The majority of traumatic brain injuries sustained by members of the US Armed Forces are classified as mild TBI, also known as concussion."[*]

The theory Hilchey and Pomaville were working on was that several of the most common symptoms related to TBI were at the root of preventing these veterans from succeeding in an academic setting. As we've touched on previously, and General Laich wrote about in his book, many of our heroes answer the call of duty as a way out of poverty, and as a way to ultimately further their education, both through direct military-related training but

---

[*] These statistics are contested as a variety of sources report numbers that range from as low as 50,000 to as high as 400,000 (Rand Corporation).

also through post-service college courses. The GI Bill provides significant educational opportunities and in today's competitive job market, succeeding in academics after service may mean the difference between becoming a productive member of civilian society or another statistic.

Through the Academic Prep Group modeling exercises, Hilchey and Pomaville discovered that peer feedback and support was a key factor in the rehabilitation process, and that integrating veterans who were farther along in their TBI recovery with those just starting out created a healthy peer learning environment that resulted in 73 percent of participants saying that the strategies they'd learned through the group had provided them the skills and confidence to continue their education and succeed. In follow-up interviews, 100 percent of these veterans stated that the integration of technology-based learning and help with navigating disability services offered at all colleges and universities helped significantly to improve their academic experience.

"I did my research on this new generation of TBI and PTSD patients. As a therapist, I looked for what was most functional, what would make the most difference because these men and women are so young and have a whole lifetime to deal with this. I wanted to get them back out and about, back into the community, back to their families, their lives," Hilchey said.

Not unlike the slow, deliberate pace of medicine and therapy changes undertaken in research and treatment of TBI patients such as me, Hilchey designed various treatment materials grouped together such as memory tasks, attention tasks, sequencing, etc.

"I pretty much tailored the treatment to fit my patient's cognitive level and needs," Hilchey said. "After a few years of this,

I was sent to the annual VA TBI conference where I discovered that an interdisciplinary team from the Boston, Portland, and San Diego VA systems had developed this fabulous program called CogSMART, which is available online.[37] It was essentially everything I had piecemealed together into one six-week program, created for a group setting. I adopted the program but tweaked it to fit the needs of my veterans and limitations of our resources."

My faith in medical science to help me rehabilitate and recover was not misplaced, but I was still far from normal. I kept faking my way through my days, working half-days as much as possible, and seeing only one patient per hour instead of three. Like a majority of TBI sufferers, I continued to have problems with finding the right word, but I was able to speak in simple sentences and get the point across. Unfortunately, this change from being very conversational to somewhat short (by necessity) both concerned and bothered my patients. Some were even angered, at times, as if I were ignoring them on purpose. I was, after all, being sought as a care giver, not a care taker.

I was still unable to drive, read well, or work a full day, but like a lighthouse in the distance, I found every now and then throughout my day a wave of energy, like a beam of light, would sweep across my brain and give me a sense of renewal. I was seeing patients for four to five hours a day by now. My fatigue had lessened and I was beginning to tolerate lighting by having the fluorescent lights removed and using incandescent lamps with a dimmer switch installed instead. One important strategy for recovery is controlling what you can; the dimmer switch allowed me a more precise tweak to whatever light level I could tolerate on a given day. At this point in recovery I was tweaking my environment to tolerate the new me as much as I could to help the new me tolerate my environment.

CHAPTER SIX

AN APPLE A DAY

My day of reckoning arrived six weeks into my stalled recovery. By this point it was mid-January and in Ohio that means the long, dark days of winter cast the world in a brown-grey shadow void of any semblance of the joyous colors found in spring and summer. In my previous life I would've been so consumed by my work that the lack of sunny distractions was almost welcome, but now I would give anything to be able to dance on a partly sunny hillside singing like Julie Andrews in *The Sound of Music*. Instead of dancing and singing my brain remained in revolt, leaving so much of my life consumed only with thoughts of myself. I was trapped within my own mind, unable to make my brain function so that I might even just express myself as I had my whole life.

I hated what I'd been reduced to.

I hated the symptoms I was experiencing.

I hated my brain for constantly processing all of my symptoms, issues, what-ifs, and so on.

I hated being tired all the time—I'd never rested so much in my life, so why hadn't my brain healed by now? My CT scan said I was normal, so why did I feel so many miles, no, so many lifetimes away from what I knew to be normal?

With each dose of amantadine, I realized that the drug was like a battery losing its charge. As the last dose slowly dissipated from my system my brain slowed to a halt until my next dose. I'd found that caffeine and chocolate provided small boosts to the amantadine effect, but ultimately it wasn't me and it wasn't my resting that was in charge of my brain function—my brain was dependent on some chemical interaction that it was no longer creating on its own.

For all of my talk about faith in medical science in the previous chapter, I was alone, no family living nearby or able to relocate for me and an occasional friend or colleague as my only outlet from the darkness of my private thoughts. During one of my daily cab rides home I began considering how exposed I had become: all these strangers driving me to and from my house. They knew I lived alone. Strangers who knew I had a disability and was well-employed. I felt as though I was becoming a target for possible harm. When I got inside my house I felt anxiety. The answering machine light was blinking at me so I went to it, looking forward to the possibility of some small connection to another person whom I knew.

The machine functioned perfectly, provided me with just what I'd wanted to hear, but my brain was unable to concentrate on and process what was being said. I found I was unable to filter the information and focus. I could not remember the number. I had to write it down. After almost a dozen times of listening and re-listening to the message I was finally able to write down the phone number, one number at a time. I was not much better than I had been shortly after my first dose of amantadine, and that reality check meant to me that I had lost my mind—a sentiment later re-defined by one of my colleagues, that I hadn't lost my mind but I had lost my brain.

For so many people suffering from TBI there is an obvious difficulty with filtering what they are saying or doing—their outward expressions—but what is less obvious to most people is how difficult filtering the incoming information is as well.

Night was falling and the darkness swept in, both externally and internally with that stupid phone still sitting there, mocking me. No matter how long I stared at that simple device I couldn't remember a phone number to save my life; and what I needed now more than ever was a life saver.

"Get busy living, or get busy dying," Morgan Freeman's character, Red, says in the film *Shawshank Redemption*, somewhat ironically after mentioning to the character Andy that, "to get what you want on the outside, you just use the Yellow Pages."[38] Well, in this emotional state what I wanted was to get outside of my brain, and I couldn't use the Yellow Pages for that even if they'd have helped. So instead of getting busy living, I gave a cold dark look at getting busy dying.

How could I continue this way? How could I continue doctoring? How could I take care of anyone else when I couldn't take care of myself? If I cannot read. If I cannot retain knowledge. If I cannot balance a checkbook or even write a check. If I do not ever get any better than this, well, how could I go on? I am here to serve. I am not here to be a burden. Without that ability to care for myself and others, my reason for existing no longer existed.

In working with our veterans, I understand this feeling of being a burden. Many veterans suffering from a TBI feel this way, whether or not they act upon it. One of the worst parts of my consideration of committing suicide is that at the time my brain was so scrambled I could not even think of a way to do it. This is key, because this is ultimately what saved my life in that moment. This is not the case for our military members, and even first responders like police or firefighters, also there to serve. All of these professions are well-versed in using firearms and other lethal methods—often with those tools at hand. These souls with battered brains do not impose a pause like I had. As Dr. Joiner stated, regarding the three requirements for suicide (desire, ability, and feeling of burdensomeness), at that very dark moment I lacked ability, and that made all the difference. The hopelessness and the burdensomeness I was experiencing was put on pause for just a moment—and that momentary pause was from my flicker of faith, which was enough to get me to this point—where I am telling you this story instead of being eulogized.

Staff Sgt. Armstrong began welling up when he talked about this in our interview. "By this time I had served nine years in the Army and I knew my career was done. I couldn't be effective anymore because of my TBI. My family, like my brothers and sisters and my mom, they all thought my job was awesome—but they didn't know about my actual work, about my deployments and my injuries.

"So when I was dealing with my injuries and struggling to go through the process with the VA to get things covered, and trying to go to school, and trying to see my kids, and work, well, my brain couldn't handle it all and I broke down. It's like I needed a prosthetic but there's no prosthetic for the brain; and my family didn't understand.

"They looked at me like, 'Are you just getting ornery or are you getting old or what?' They thought I could just take a pill and get better, and so I told them like, 'yeah, I think I can try that', even though I knew there wasn't a pill that was going to fix this. I'd been on dozens of pills and none of them fixed this. I didn't want to let them down, and I didn't want to be a burden to them, so it was like coming home wasn't really what you think coming home should be. I was trying to protect them and it meant I didn't have anyone I could talk to about this," Armstrong said.

Both Sgt. Guillermo and retired Marine Sgt. Chris Lawrence, who also suffers a TBI, said the same thing in interviews: that you couldn't show injuries in the military and that when you got home, the stigma wasn't really any better.

"Obviously this is a testosterone driven MOS [military occupational specialty] and your whole job of jumping out of a plane and killing the bad guy means you have to compartmentalize what you've seen, but the stigma that goes with, especially PTSD in a combat unit, prohibits promotion and everything else because you are looked at as weak, or crazy," Guillermo said. "For us it was like that, where we had to hide our concerns and for some guys that meant doing drugs or some other way out."

My thoughts of suicide were, in reality, a survival mechanism. I spent four cold hours sitting in the dark, on the kitchen floor, developing a plan for an out—an exit strategy in case this got worse. Again, it was ironic that before the injury, I could have discussed about ten ways to take my life effectively, given my ER training. However, here I was, struggling to think of even one. It was my saving grace that it took so long. Yet, knowing this was an option actually allowed me to put that aside and begin to focus on what to do next. I gave myself eight to ten weeks tops to "get busy living" and if that didn't work then I would reconsider my exit. I actually came up with a very solid exit plan, after those four hours, but I do not want to share that with my readers. What I want to share, instead, is this: PAUSE! It makes a difference between light and dark, between life and death—literally.

Looking up at the counter from where I sat I saw my Apple Macintosh sitting there in front of me. Like dealing with a computer that gets locked up, I began considering the idea of trying to reboot my brain. This was an older desktop model, an LC, with the built-in screen and lovely little smiley face icon that welcomed me during boot-up. Even after hitting an all-time low over my inability to use a telephone, I somehow saw my Mac as my best option for rehabilitation and rebooting my brain.

I got off the floor and dusted myself off, deciding that like a system update, I needed to download everything I'd forgotten into my brain, and let it reboot with the new information. It was about 8 p.m. that evening when my rehabilitation started in earnest.

Like those veterans who have participated in the modeling under Hilchey, or those using the CogSMART method, technology would play a crucial role in my return to a productive life. The very first thing I attempted on the computer was to find the text of the "Gettysburg Address" online. This short speech I'd memorized as an eight-year-old seemed like as good a place to start as any, although when I looked at it now it seemed to just be gibberish. Thank heavens for the Apple's built-in intuitiveness. It was most helpful, especially considering my first attempts at spelling "Gettysburg."

As I've mentioned, my motor skills were still not very good, and TBI commonly presents challenges with a sufferer's vision, particularly related to staring at a flickering computer monitor. The quiver of light and the reflections gave me headaches and eye pain. I had a mission though, and so I typed slowly away, reading haltingly but reading, and kept myself moving forward. No matter how much of that speech sounded like gibberish to me, I clung to the one phrase that had stuck with me through all of this: "Four score and seven years ago."

Prior to my TBI I could sit for six hours studying, never moving except to go on to the next page, memorizing one after another. Now I spent as much time looking away from the screen as I did looking at the screen, forcing myself to sit there for as long as I could and resisting the urge to wander off for water or some other break. I managed to work like this for a few hours at a time even though my concentration floated all over the place.

The most difficult times were when the computer would freeze up trying to load something. In those moments it was easy for me to lose patience with what I was doing, or to lose track of what I was waiting for. Given that this was the era of dial-up internet access, computer freeze was something I dealt with often. Fortunately for me I've always subscribed to the concept of *no-pain, no-gain,* and my determination to recover was growing stronger with each new page load. With the computer on the kitchen counter, I would continue to force-feed my brain until it became nice and plump once again.

In the beginning I just wanted to read and relearn how to use words when I was speaking so that I would no longer sound so childish and simple. Eventually that grew tedious because while my reading was improving my speech was not advancing by much, so I decided to attempt mathematics. My colleagues had told me over and over that my injury must be in my left-brain since my speech and logic skills were suffering along with the numbness on the right half of my body. Due to this, it made sense I would have lost my arithmetic skills as well and I dearly wanted them back. I pulled up the calculator application and like a grade school child I began with some very basic addition, then moved on to subtraction, multiplication, and finally division. I have never gone back and tried to retrieve my algebraic or calculus skills, of which I mourn the loss. Eventually I moved on to trying to understand geography, but that was a disaster.

Medical science is rife with disasters that become discoveries though, and this geography experiment began leading me toward a theory that has been further fleshed out by some in the TBI research community. I was never good at geography in the first place, and as I mentioned earlier, I had suffered from topographagnosia, making my spatial awareness that much worse. Emerging from all of this is the theory that a TBI can cause the loss of many of our brain's capabilities but included in that loss may also be the inability to learn new things that had not been well-enforced, or known at all, prior to the injury.

Years later, I would be fortunate enough to meet Michael Lipton, MD, PhD, a neuroradiologist and researcher at the Albert Einstein College of Medicine, who explained to me that by overworking those parts of the brain which were not damaged, such as how I was engaging (albeit with some difficulty) my reading and writing center, a TBI sufferer will continue to strengthen the healthy brain tissue while allowing time for the bad connections to lay down new pathways—which led to this "rebooting" that I was looking for. I had never in my life written lyrically prior to my TBI, but I began experimenting with songs and poems because it was the part of my brain that was working, and I thought I'd better press on with what little I felt I could accomplish.

In researching diagnostic techniques for TBI, partially in conjunction with the Resurrecting Lives Foundation, Lipton demonstrated that using diffusion tensor imaging (DTI) to map brain abnormalities related to TBI was effective in detecting the subtle changes so frequently missed by MRI and CT.[39] This process works by tracing the uniformity of movement of water molecules through brain tissue. According to Lipton, the axons in the brain connect cells like the cabling in a computer network. When these axons are healthy, water moves with the orientation of the axon, but is constrained from movement across the axon. Damage to or loss of axons leads to less uniform movement of water, detected as low fractional anisotropy, or Low FA.

In speaking with Lipton, he explained the hypothesis that higher FA, also seen in TBI patients, reflects "supranormal" organization and may indicate a "response where the brain is trying to compensate for the injury." Under this hypothesis, if the theory holds, then by utilizing the newer DTI testing instead of the CT or MRI testing, doctors should be able to identify what regions of the brain have suffered damage, and where the brain is attempting to compensate for the damage, and then develop a therapy plan around reinforcement of healthy axons as a way to compensate for lost network function.

"We use the imaging, but we're also interested in genetic factors and other medical co-morbidities when trying to determine a risk profile," Lipton said. "The problem with treating everyone who has potentially suffered a mild TBI is that about 70 percent of them will recover completely on their own. So right now we don't know (if you have a concussion) if you'll be part of the 70 percent that recovers on their own, or the 30 percent that won't. This means it is impractical to treat everyone because then you don't know for certain that a treatment worked, or maybe it is just that the patient is in the majority group. This is why our work to identify a profile of who won't get better on their own is a big step forward in ultimately determining treatment plans.

"There is this desire to come up with a one-size-fits-all solution, and one that can treat the patient rapidly, but we need to think differently about what is happening and how to treat it," he said. "For example, an outright ban of soccer headers for children and young teens up to, say, 14 years old may decrease mild TBI in that age category, but will we then see a spike in 15-year-olds who don't know how to properly head the ball? Does repeated heading have the same negative impact on every player who does it? This is what we need to nail down first, because we certainly should not be telling people just to stay inside and avoid anything that might possibly cause an injury of any kind."

Apple's "Think Different" campaign premiered just before my injury, and, to this day I find it amusing that I owe so much of my thinking differently about brain rehab to my Apple computer. As I regained more and more of my ability to communicate through writing, thanks to the benefit of printing out what I typed instead of relying solely on my shaky handwriting, I even sent off a thank you letter to Steve Jobs letting him know I owed him for giving me back my brain. Since this whole experience I've been a walking advertisement for their products, always selecting their computers, phones, and now iPad over any competitor. I'm apt to say that, "an Apple a day" has a whole new meaning in my life. Technology has played a major role in returning TBI patients to their more functional selves, and the more intuitive a product the more likely it is to be beneficial to TBI patients in need of help. In fact, recently, the iPad has shown how even autistic children seem drawn to the intuitiveness of Apple products as a means of unlocking worlds and opening communication.

One of the lessons learned in Hilchey's modeling project was that "incorporating the benefits and use of technology in the classroom has improved motivation to participate in the group and to try and go back to school." The amount of consumer technology available that is beneficial to TBI sufferers such as me is staggering—brain blowing even. The use of calendar reminders on smartphones and now smart watches can relieve the strain over short-term memory loss. Additionally, technology such as *IFTTT* (*If This Then That*) can enable the sending of a wide variety of reminders or alerts based on a similarly wide variety of inputs. For example, if your smartphone detects that you left work it might remind you to stop for groceries on the way home, or alert a family member that you're on your way.

Staff Sgt. Armstrong explained that he prefers to use the speech-to-text functions of his phone and other devices due to the frustration he has when trying to manipulate small keypads. He further explained how his use of reminders and lists on his iPhone have helped make him much more reliable because he doesn't have to count on only his brain for memory. Similarly, as mentioned previously, he relies heavily on his GPS, as do I.

The mapping center of the brain is very small, only about the size of a dime, and very vulnerable to injury due to its placement in the brain. Thus, as stated earlier, one of the hallmarks of TBI is losing mapping skills. Identifying this in our returning heroes such as Armstrong is relatively easy: when a military navigator managed to find their way around the battlefields of Iraq prior to an IED blast or similarly injurious situation, but then can't navigate the small Ohio town they lived in for years before shipping out, that's an obvious sign.

I never had many navigational nor spatial skills, but I could read a map if I had to, prior to my TBI. After that, all I saw was squiggly lines and indecipherable information. For 15 years following my injury that was all I could make of a map. Then one evening, I had gotten off track and found myself at dusk in an unfamiliar and somewhat threatening-looking neighborhood. I was trying to navigate to a veterans' event but a detour—something most people would be able to just follow—threw me for a loop. Of course, Siri would choose that place and time to be "unable to assist at this time." Sitting at a stoplight that felt as though it would never change, my heart rate began to increase and my adrenaline kicked in. I grabbed the map I had with me not so much because I thought I would be able to read it, but more just to feel as if I were being proactive. With that rush of adrenaline to my brain, though, I looked and there it was—not squiggles, but decipherable lines—it was truly a map and I could read it. I've been reading them ever since.

The takeaway for me from this experience that I cannot stress enough is that, even 15 years after my injury, I recovered this part of my brain seemingly all of a sudden. Even as I write this book, more than 20 years since my injury, I am still recovering bits and pieces. For example, I went grocery shopping recently and forgot my shopping list at home. For the first time since my accident I managed to remember every item on the list—something that I hadn't been able to do even once before since the accident.

App maker Always Get Home created the self-titled iPhone app *Always Get Home* which they've made as a free download.[40] Gregory Welteroth, Jr and Steve Rockwell, who are behind the app's creation, said that the original intention was to develop an application that would help our returning veterans (and others) who have suffered from TBI and brain disease-related mapping center losses. While there are many applications that are helpful for the everyday life of all users, only certain applications cut through the complexity to provide only the essential services. For someone like myself this straight-forward approach is the only way I am able to function.

For well-meaning caregivers suggesting to a TBI sufferer that they just use an app meant for the mass public, please understand that these can be frustrating to us. Even if we're given explicit instructions for a more complex technological solution, not unlike my detour through a bad neighborhood, any number of small technological detours that would seem obvious to the regular person can completely lock up someone suffering from a TBI.

Researchers at the Institute for Creative Technologies, University of Southern California, presented work they had completed using the widely available *Microsoft Kinect Sensor* to the IEEE Engineering in Medicine and Biology Society.[41] They study TBI and patients with other neurological disorders to see if using the inexpensive technology would be beneficial in helping to regain motor control and balance based on easily repeated therapy that can be completed at home, and provide constant evaluative data to both the patient and the therapist via networked connectivity. Similarly, researchers in Brazil at the Federal University of Pernambuco, Physiotherapy Department, Applied Neuroscience Lab completed similar research confirming that, not unlike injuries requiring straight-forward physiotherapy, the use of widely-available technology that mimics specific therapies—both physical and neurological—may eliminate the necessity for patients to make specific appointments which may include travel arrangements, etc.[42]

In the Brazilian research paper, the researchers echoed the findings of therapists Hilchey and Pomaville as well as my own experience, that without the motivation and engagement of the patient, recovery is impossible. The researchers wrote, "It has been acknowledged that the efficacy of long-time treatments is highly dependent on the engagement of the patient. Health professionals are always searching for a more effective treatment that focuses not only at the elimination of the pathology symptoms but also holds the patient involved to it during the entire treatment in order to achieve the cure. The importance of taking into consideration related human factors, such as patient satisfaction and motivation is the key to ensure patient involvement and to achieve a successful treatment."

In an article titled "Video Games Show Promise as Therapy," written for Military.com, Steve Wilson of the Disabled American Veterans (DAV) explored how new video game technology is being used specifically for therapy, and particularly how first-person-shooter games like *Call of Duty* and *Medal of Honor* are a way for veterans and their families to tell the story of their experiences through a different medium, where it might open up new opportunities for therapeutic discussion.[43]

Kathleen M. Chard, PhD, is the director of the Trauma Recovery Center at the Cincinnati VA Medical Center and Professor of Psychiatry and Behavioral Neuroscience at the University of Cincinnati. She is working with TBI and PTSD patients using what she calls Virtual Reality Exposure (VRE) therapy. In this she uses a fully immersive experience that includes not just sights and sounds, but includes smells such as that of cordite and street markets.

"The VRE treatment allows us to trigger memories about the event to obtain the full story," Chard said in her interview with Wilson. "Once these memories are triggered, we can challenge those misperceptions in the veteran's mind, including areas where they may be blaming themselves for things they could not have controlled or predicted."

Video game designer Jane McGonigal gave a *TEDGlobal* presentation in 2012 where she explained how her mTBI left her with "nonstop headaches, nausea, vertigo, memory loss, mental fog."[44] After being told by her physician to rest her brain and body, to remove all stimulation, she began to lose her reason to live. Just over a month into her "rest" she explained her suicidal ideations had become "so persuasive" that she truly feared for her life; at this point she said, "I am either going to kill myself or I'm going to turn this into a game."

Initially McGonigal called her game *Jane the Concussion Slayer* and it wasn't exactly a video game at this point, more just a thought experiment played out with her sister, husband, and a few friends. By using gamification of tasks to boost her wellbeing, McGonigal found herself improving in her recovery as opposed to "resting" and sinking deeper into depression. Ultimately, having used herself as the beta tester, she launched what is now known as *SuperBetter*[45] as an iPhone and Android app aimed at providing others the same sort of gamification of recovery that she utilized.

A simple Google search will return any number of technology-based therapies being researched. One of the more successful applications of technology as therapy for those suffering TBI as well as other neurological disorders is Dr. Tej Tadi's *MindMaze*[46] application. In fact, Tadi's application has been called a "unicorn" in the technology investment arena for netting over $1 billion to further develop the already successful technology. This virtual reality simulation got its start by taking advantage of the Google Glass technology and other similar tech solutions to trick the brain into thinking it knows something that it has forgotten. As Tadi says when talking about *MindMaze*, it "tricks the brain into rewiring itself."

I invite every veteran reading this book to go to YouTube and view the Steve Jobs-narrated Apple commercial dubbed "The Crazy Ones" from the "Think Different" campaign.[47] I believe if you are reading this text and dealing with these issues then you are definitely crazy enough to think that we, all of us together, can and will change the military separation process to allow all our veterans and their families, to thrive in the civilian world.

To this day I still use my Apple computers as a primary therapy for myself. I challenge myself to attempt to lay down some new bit of knowledge each day—even if it was once something I'd have considered old news—and what has come of this has been way beyond my expectations. As I've said before, "an Apple a day" can be more than just a cliché!

CHAPTER SEVEN

CIRCUITS LAY DOWN

For six weeks, for at least four hours a day every single day, I forced myself to sit in front of that Apple computer and attempt to read, calculate, problem solve, whatever I could, but still I felt as though I was getting nowhere. Was I laying down new circuits or was I wasting my time? That seemed like a completely unanswerable inquiry at this point in my recovery. Every morning I'd sit myself back down at the computer and every morning I'd realize I hadn't retained anything from what I'd done the day before. The only thing that I remembered was how I used to know all of this stuff and now I didn't. By this point I had experienced one very important lesson: the all-or-nothing phenomenon.

All-or-nothing as in I couldn't speak until I could, there was no half step; I saw with blurred double vision until I didn't, there was no partial deglazing; and now I was placing my faith in this phenomenon happening once more with my intellect.

I have always loved competition, and Olympic diving is no exception. The sport has fascinated me since my earliest memories of watching ABC's weekend *Wide World of Sports* broadcasts. My scientific mind has always dazzled over how the divers utilize so much brute strength, while managing to appear graceful as they make these aerial gymnastics seem effortless. Long before my accident, when I was completing my training to work as a rehabilitation therapist, I had drilled into my practice the words of multiple gold medalist Greg Louganis: "Repetition, repetition, repetition." Louganis said that his massive success was only because of his tenacity and commitment; any God-given talents he had would mean nothing without this constant, repetitive practice. In our current era of research, including Malcom Gladwell's *Outliers*[48] (and similar studies about how repetition is as important to success as just about anything else), this doesn't seem so revolutionary, but having learned that lesson so early in my life, well ahead of the 10,000-hours principle, I was instinctively able to cling to the idea like a lifeline.

Part of understanding TBI is understanding that similar impacts to the head may result in drastically different outcomes in different people. In an ironic twist of fate, Louganis himself had suffered a serious blow to his head in the 1988 Seoul Olympics. During a preliminary round of the springboard competition his head struck the board. Whereas the force of his impact and mine had likely been similar, both of us suffering a TBI, he managed to continue on in the competition and win gold yet again—ultimately earning ABC's *Wide World of Sports* "1988 Athlete of the Year" award—whereas I'm forever waiting to win my first gold medal equivalent at anything. Having precious little natural athleticism before and after my TBI, I was not frustrated by lack of physical coordination.

This similar impact but different brain injury and effect on the patient is exactly what the researchers at Albert Einstein College of Medicine, completing the previously-mentioned study directed by Dr. Lipton, meant in regard to the roughly 70 percent of mTBI sufferers ultimately healing themselves. For me, I needed to embrace the compensatory response the way I was embracing repetition. The research using DTI even shows there are clear signs of the difference from one mTBI patient to the next. With help from the Resurrecting Lives Foundation, Lipton's team was able to study 16 veterans who had suffered mTBI in blast incidents alongside a control group of their siblings, who had no diagnosis of TBI.[49] In the findings the team wrote that, "The uniformity of diffusion direction—an indicator of whether tissue has maintained its microstructural integrity—is measured as fractional anisotropy (FA), on a zero-to-one scale. In the latest study, areas of abnormally low FA (reflecting abnormal brain regions) were observed in concussion patients but not in controls. Each concussion patient had a unique spatial pattern of low FA that evolved over the study period."

I had trusted fully in repetition earlier in my life in order to become the competent and trusted physician I'd become, and all joking aside, while I know there is no gold medal for that, I desperately wanted to return myself to that status. There was no way I would give up my faith in this formula now. Tenacity had become my instinct and this is one of the keys to rehabilitation, not only for the person suffering the TBI but also for the caregivers. The effects of a TBI don't take holidays and neither can the work required to recover.

I had surpassed the eight-week mark since my injury at this point, and it had been six weeks since my initial bump in rehabilitation that I'd received from the amantadine. At five weeks into this whole process, I had another instant recovery—the last of them prior to this period.

Since the injury, I had not had normal sensation on the right side of my body. All I had been left with was the ability to feel some pressure changes, but not much, and I felt no environmental changes. A hot shower meant nothing to the right side of my body. Hot or cold, I was indifferent, until one morning when I went to shower and things had clearly changed. The water pelting my right side seemed painful—like I was caught in a hailstorm and being pelted repeatedly with tiny balls of ice. At first I was startled by the experience and somewhat instinctively tried adjusting the flow but to no avail. The feeling was so intense that I decided to rush my shower and get the heck out of there. That was when something fascinating happened. In the course of a few minutes I went from painful pelts to a burning sensation to voila!—the return of my temperature sensation! No longer did I feel as though I was being pelted. Instead I felt the light, soothing water pressure, and it was warm water. Two sensations had returned: touch and temperature, which I had not experienced since the injury. A new pathway had been created and I've never returned to that anesthetic state.

If it hadn't been for these small victories I may not have made it this far, and even still I was not anywhere near done with my fight. I gave myself another four weeks to show significantly more signs of recovery or else I would again consider my exit plan.

Each day, following my four-hour consumption of information off the internet, I would then sit and free-form write. I had never done this sort of thing before. I was a woman of science and as much as I could enjoy the arts, they weren't previously a part of my practice. Knowing that fact was extremely helpful to me however, because it allowed me to remove the critical lens through which I was looking at myself in regard to what had gone missing for me—the historical data, the arithmetic skill, the logic-forward problem solving. I beat myself up over my inability to do the simplest division and multiplication, and reading scientific papers was frustrating me to no end. So I decided that my new brain, which seemed to enjoy writing poetry and song lyrics, was taking over. My assumption was that if neural rehabilitation works for regaining physical control, balance, and other motor skills, then why couldn't it work for cognition? Functionally this was the practice of neuroplasticity before it had been given that name.

Research is still in infancy regarding specific prescription drugs and dietary changes that truly impact either cognitive or functional recovery from TBI, but there is plenty of evidence that enhancing dopamine levels tends to speed up the rebuilding and reconnecting of your brain's circuitry. Drugs that fall into this category include things like amantadine, methylphenidate, and modafinil to name just a few—but not unlike the application of psychotropic drugs for mental illness, any use of drugs for the rehabilitation of a TBI patient must be properly titrated by a physician who is willing to play chess against the condition. This is a long-term, close-contact component of rehabilitation with extensive individualization to each person.

The desire to return to normal is exactly why self-medication is so common for our patients suffering from TBI or PTSD. Unfortunately, with no real gold standard protocol in place for treatment and only 8-10 percent of physicians trained in TBI recovery, our injured veterans find little recourse other than to rely on the medicinal crutches offered to them. A patient with a TBI will attempt to jump start his or her brain with caffeine, nicotine, amphetamines, or cocaine, or dull their senses with alcohol, marijuana, and opiates. There is no injury that leads to a more rapid demise than TBI. The downward spiral of co-morbidities is swift and non-forgiving, leading to substance abuse, unemployment, homelessness, incarceration, and suicide. Women in the military who suffer from TBI may have done so in combat zones or as a result of military sexual trauma, all of which have many psychosocial impediments to recovery. Truly, we must do more to rapidly diagnose and treat each TBI patient on an individual basis.

"I've been through four primary care doctors in the three years since I'd finally gotten my diagnosis because they kept dropping me. They didn't know what to do and I felt like I wasn't getting anywhere," Staff Sgt. Armstrong said. Besides his TBI and PTSD, Armstrong's spine was injured in the blast and still causes him regular pain.

"Because I wasn't able to get my rating increased with the VA until recently, I wasn't able to get any sort of effective help for my pain, even just the pain related to my back and neck, much less for my headaches," Armstrong said. "So everything I've been doing has mostly been frowned upon. I was going to the gym, thinking that would help with calming my anxiety and lowering my stress levels since I couldn't work anymore, and now I'm officially considered unemployable. I had the time; but it was causing me too much physical pain. The MRI of my back shows what a mess it is. I still enjoy hiking and other outdoor activities, just lower impact stuff."

For Armstrong, who lives in a medical marijuana state, and knows a friend who received relief from his painful war injuries through this use, this may be a possible option in the future. However, many health care providers, myself included, are awaiting the results of controlled studies on this treatment before sanctioning the recommendation.

Like many of his fellow veterans, Armstrong ran afoul of the law due to alcohol, getting his first and only DUI not long after returning state-side. Fortunately for him, this took place in Ohio where one of the very first veteran courts had been set up, and this is where I initially met him.

"I'd never done anything like that before," Armstrong said. "Before coming back I would've never let myself drink past the legal limit and then drive, and I guess I just hadn't paid attention and I think I figured at the time that if I could drive a Humvee safely through Baghdad I could easily get my buddy and I home safely in Mansfield. I still feel ashamed about that."

Ask any ER doctor and he or she will relate the negative effects of alcohol dealt with every weekend, regardless of TBI. The fact that it is essentially a legal over-the-counter medicine without any clearly redeeming qualities makes it so much worse. For being so easy to obtain, it is also, in my opinion, one of the worst of the self-medications because of how it tends to increase depression, anger, and even violence in its users. Alcohol further disconnects the executive functioning of the brain, further impairing judgment, further threatening safety to the users and those who come in contact with them.

In a study completed by the Ohio Valley Center for Brain Injury Prevention and Rehabilitation, part of The Ohio State University Wexner Medical Center, researchers found that the symptoms associated with a TBI closely mimic the effects of alcohol, such as loss of balance, reduced motor skills, and lowered inhibitions.[50] On the basis of that alone, alcohol use following a TBI will then only increase those issues and present an increased likelihood for additional TBI to occur. Each successive TBI then has a cumulative effect as we've discussed previously, leading to ever-increasing symptoms and increasing the risk for CTE and other ailments associated with the brain.

Worse still is the suggestion from the research by Charles H. Bombardier, PhD, and Aaron Turner, PhD, (et al) that alcohol has an "additive effect on brain structure and function" in relation to how the healing process takes place in an injured brain.[51] According to the research, it is believed that alcohol decreases the brain's ability to rebuild injured pathways and hampers the brain's ability to build new neural pathways around the TBI-affected areas. Beyond limitations to recovery, or completely stalling recovery, alcohol can also cause excessive damage: sufferers of a TBI are already at a higher risk for seizure than the general public and alcohol use "lowers the seizure threshold and may trigger seizures."

Finally, regarding alcohol, its use in combination with prescribed medication can have significant effect on how medication interacts with the body, including the negation of effects or the introduction of serious and even life-threatening drug interactions. Of those medications prescribed by physicians, opiates are second on the list for introducing serious problems for TBI patients—especially when mixed with alcohol.

Opiate addiction is one of the fastest growing drug addictions in the US and is often traced back to the legitimate prescription of opioids such as oxycodone and oxycodone with acetaminophen. Without close supervision, that legitimate prescription can quickly lead to abuse. The mixture of opioids and alcohol specifically have caused a significant number of fatal overdoses in the US and in particular within this age demographic. In many cases these fatalities may be masking the actual number of suicides taking place within the broader community of veterans and military personnel as well as specifically within that of TBI and PTSD sufferers.

One of the difficulties faced by individuals such as Staff Sgt. Armstrong is the fact that he isn't able to work a regular, full-time job, but he is able to work unstructured schedules, such as part-time security or private investigation duties. In many cases those positions require that the employee retain a weapons classification such as Concealed Carry (CCW). Those classifications currently preclude the licensee from also utilizing medical marijuana in many states that have legalized marijuana in medicinal form.

"Part of the struggle is that all of my friends have regular jobs so I have to keep myself busy during the day, but there's not much to do and no one else to spend time with," Armstrong said. "Marijuana may take away a lot of pain and headaches, and cut down on anxiety, but you can only do it in the evenings if you want to be productive during the day. For a lot of guys though, there's just nothing to do, so they do that."

The debate over medical marijuana continues in most states, with only a handful legalizing the practice and fewer still making marijuana legal across the board. As much as I understand just how controversial the use of marijuana is, I have seen several of my TBI patients who are using medical marijuana appropriately as medicine appear to have significantly decreased the effects of migraines and anxiety. It appears that marijuana may not affect executive function the same way that alcohol does, but more research is forthcoming on this use for TBI.

For my personal experience, anecdotally at least, stimulants such as caffeine, chocolate, and some "energy drinks" have had the most effect in helping to bring back some spark of light to my life. That being said, I would never advocate for the use of stimulants such as speed and cocaine as they have addictive and destructive properties. The amantadine that helped to wake up my brain and speed its recovery is a good example of a dopamine enhancer, helping to stimulate brain cells in the hopes that they reconnect the damaged circuits. The fact remains that more research must be done to provide a more specific prescription for medicinal treatment of TBI.

All of which is to say that while there is a desperate need for more research into TBI treatment and the development of appropriate diagnostic, treatment, and prescription protocols, there are steps in place currently that can be taken. Caregivers are crucial at this step because, as I've said above, self-medication often leads to serious setbacks. Without a support system in place setbacks are guaranteed. Included in the Resource section of this book is a guide for "Professionals Working with Persons with TBI."[52] I would like to preface this resource by saying any caregiver serving a TBI patient is holding a full-time job and may as well consider themselves a "professional."

The guide was originally intended to help physicians and therapists understand the special accommodations necessary when working with a TBI patient, but those same sorts of accommodations fit in nearly every setting. Often in our society we look at something referred to as an accommodation as a sort of luxury, entitlement, or special treatment. What we are talking about though, plain and simple, is clearing a path to focus energy on recovering the functionality of the brain instead of fixating on how bright the lights are or how stressful grocery shopping might be.

This struggle was echoed in interviews with several other soldiers, including Sgt. Lawrence who was injured when insurgents blew up a bridge he and his staff sergeant had been crossing. Besides losing his lower leg in the explosion, he was given a post-traumatic stress diagnosis—but not a TBI diagnosis.

"They spent six months putting me back together and then another eight months rehabbing me while I participated in the Wounded Warrior Battalion," Lawrence said; the WWB is internal to the Marines, giving wounded soldiers a place to continue their service even though it isn't in a battlefield position. "I think it helped in regard to my recovery because I was still able to fulfill some role while trying to figure out what my future would be since I couldn't be a soldier anymore. I spent about two years counseling other wounded soldiers until funding for that got cut and now I'm going through the police academy unsponsored."

Lawrence said that getting a VA rating (diagnosis-related benefits) for PTSD is a catch 22—one that he doesn't feel is worth it.

"I didn't seek the diagnosis but they gave it to me anyway. Now it is causing me problems trying to get into police duty," Lawrence said. "The stigma of PTSD and TBI creates a catch 22. Like when

I was injured my staff sergeant was, too, but he didn't have any obvious injuries. However he could barely walk or talk so he got shunned by the rest of the company and made fun of a lot which caused him problems with his military career.

"I remember when I came back to the States and news crews would try and get young Marines off base to talk about what PTSD was but our superiors told us it didn't exist and not to talk about it. Now the script has flipped but those same people are still in charge and instead when you get that rating you're treated almost worse than an abused puppy like on those ASPCA infomercials."

"Being a vet with a diagnosis or injury doesn't make you any less capable, we just need opportunities to work and become functioning members of society," Lawrence said.

Giving a TBI sufferer the time and space to sit and challenge their brain in ways similar to how I sat at my Apple and challenged myself to figure out what was lost forever and what might be discovered again is crucial to laying down circuits and rewiring the brain. The statistics are bad enough considering most of our military personnel spend an average of five to eight years post-TBI before they are accurately diagnosed. Yet all the research points to the importance of treating a TBI as soon as possible after injury for maximum recovery and rehabilitation. Fix it right and fix it immediately because once the injured and interrupted pathways have settled in rewiring becomes very difficult, indeed.

After surpassing the eight-week mark I was concerned that all of my work was for naught; each day I awoke to another clean slate which I'd fill again. However, a few more days of this regimen and I once again had that polarized charge of energy flowing through my body, not unlike when my eyes cleared up and when I could speak again. Similar to the feeling right before lightning strikes, I felt a pulse through my body as if each neuron was receiving a little extra charge. I developed a slight twitch in my right arm, the one which only weeks ago had no sensation in at all. I once again began to fear I was about to have a seizure and possibly worse yet, a stroke. My brain felt as though it was fogging over, sort of like the snow on TV when you select a channel without reception. I knew I couldn't drive myself to the hospital and I didn't think I could call the squad so I decided I would ride it out.

I went to the bedroom and lay on the floor, surrounding myself with pillows just in case I had a seizure or epileptic fit—I didn't want to add a broken neck into the mix. The twitching increased and lasted a couple of hours along with the feeling of electricity. Throughout the night I held firm that I would get through this the same as I had previous nights, with my brain, my faith in God, and my medical books at my side. The last time I remember looking at the clock it was about 11 p.m.

I drifted off to sleep shortly thereafter and that was when something totally amazing happened.

My brain rebooted!

It was as if I was watching a movie in fast-forward, frame after frame flying by. I watched as past learning appeared in chronological order, from the simple math from grade school, to algebra and beyond, then geography and so on, up through my university-level social studies, mathematics, science courses, etc. This lasted seemingly for hours but it is hard to say given my detached feeling from it all. I lay there still twitching, watching a version of myself with fascination, not completely sure if I was asleep or awake and not really caring either way. All night long, equations, historic dates, photos of important geographic and historical locations, poetry, philosophic phrases, all rushed through my brain, as if I were cataloging my brain's hard drive with a view master of rapidly clicking slides. I had no control over the speed, the content, nor the time allocated to this intel, but it was laid out, in chronologic order, subject specific, and it covered nearly 40 years of data.

Around 6 a.m. I became aware that I was waking up and that I was very groggy, but amazed at what I remembered occurring. I wasn't convinced that I hadn't gone completely crazy, but if that's what happened at least it was exciting. The whole event was exhausting, and I spent the rest of the day at home, having called off work, and I tried not to stress my brain any further—as if the newly re-acquired knowledge that had returned would once again disappear if I didn't leave well enough alone. My estimation was that during those several hours of the reboot I seemed to have regained about 65 percent of what I had previously known and understood prior to my TBI.

For now, my exit strategy could be thrown out the door as I had gotten much more than just my knowledge back. Lightning finally struck and with it came a flood of hope for my recovery.

CHAPTER EIGHT

REBOOT

You might think that having a breakthrough like this would warrant that I begin a lecture circuit praising the regimen for amantadine, Apple, caffeine, and the internet, but you'd be wrong. It took me years to admit my level of disability during my recovery. As relieved as I was at the prospect of finding some amount of my previously lost brain, I was equally concerned that revealing all that had just occurred might lead some of the people around me to feel vindicated in thinking I was somehow faking my injury, or that I had lost my mind. Not only in that moment, but even today I recognize that there are valid reasons for other people to think this way.

Medical science does not like what it cannot explain, and the interworking of the brain is highly suspect given the enormity of ignorance of brain function. Not for lack of trying or desire, but science has to overcome major hurdles in understanding brain function which go beyond our current scientific capabilities.

First is the specific mapping of the brain's hardware. As mentioned earlier in this book the science behind brain function for decades had been that the brain is a massive structure of neurons that fire off in a sort of binary code formation not unlike a computer, either on or off, and that series of switch settings is what leads to our consciousness. For many lay people this remains the depth of the understanding. In primary school biology class, this is what is most frequently taught with the footnote that science doesn't understand what series of switches make for what sort of "consciousness" or "decision-making" or "personality," just that the mystery happens through neurons firing on and off. This concept, sometimes referred to as the "neuron doctrine," is a controversial one because it simplifies brain function and even consciousness as only that which happens above the processing level of neurons. In other words, all of the chemical interactions and supportive cells such as the glia are not included in this theory. Even a quick Google search will lead to very reputable sources, such as the National Institute of Health's Institute on Aging report (specifically one titled "Neurons and Their Jobs"[53]) explaining brain function through the lens of the neuron doctrine. Researchers such as Dr. Lipton have found that there is so much more going on though than this on/off electrical state.

In Lipton's ongoing and substantial research, he found that the brain cell's ability to pass water molecules is directly related to functionality. Neuroscience researcher Robert Stufflebeam, PhD, who directs The Mind Project, is similarly working to not only better understand the underlying structures of neurons and transmission, but to also offer a more complete curriculum to both primary and secondary students than what the age-old neuron doctrine portrays.[54] To illustrate the complexity science faces when understanding the hardware of the brain, in a paper titled "Neurons, Synapses, Action Potentials, and Neurotransmission," Stufflebeam wrote:

> "Processing so many kinds of information requires many types of neurons; there may be as many as 10,000 types of them. Processing so much information requires a lot of neurons. How many? Well, 'best estimates' indicate that there are around 200 billion neurons in the brain alone! And as each of these neurons is connected to between 5,000 and 200,000 other neurons, the number of ways that information flows among neurons in the brain is so large, it is greater than the number of stars in the entire universe!"

As most of us are taught in our secondary school biology courses, we generally don't think of such a multitude of types of neurons, much less any attempt to conceptualize the incredible number of neural pathways constructed between neurons of similar and differing types—nor how those pathways affect our sense of self and ability to reason.

Harvard research scientist Dr. Kit Parker, Lt. Colonel in the US Air Force, and trained paratrooper, just released findings that, not unlike Lipton's discovery of using DTI to map microscopic damage to the brain, there is also a protein connector called an integrin that is sub-cell level but can be detected and used to map damaged brain tissue.[55] One additional difficulty is that cell trauma doesn't always result in dead or even visibly damaged brain cells. When interviewed by his alma mater Boston University early on about his research, Parker explained that, "The paradigm for brain injury is that the membrane of the nerve cell gets ripped open and the cell dies. But the membrane of a neuron is like the skin on a hound dog—it's floppy and not a good conduit of mechanical energy, so it doesn't always tear in trauma."

He added that, "If the cell's still alive, there's a treatment opportunity. Our ultimate goal is to identify drug targets and arm the pharmaceutical industry for the long run with a tool set for TBI drug discovery."

Of course the neural hardware is only one part of the equation—there is the software to be considered as well, which for our purpose we'll call consciousness. Consciousness for some people may not exist at all in the way human kind has generally considered it. For some scientists and philosophers, consciousness is merely the interaction of the chemicals and electrons within all living things and there is no actual choice, it is just the chaos of these information transmissions that lead to action. Ultimately it is up to those scientists and philosophers to probe for what the connection is between the hardware and the software. To pose the question in terms of this book's core metaphor—what is the connection between the mechanical process to turn on a light bulb and the experience of the light it emits?

Journalist Bob Woodruff very famously and publicly suffered his TBI in a much more traumatic fashion than I had, and he is also a champion for our heroes with TBI, publicly speaking out about how his recovery took place. Once he'd gotten past the acute injury period and come out of the coma associated with his severe brain trauma, he similarly devoted time to rehabilitating his brain the way an athlete might rehabilitate their body—repetition.

Woodruff's wife, Lee, very courageously told the story of his injury and recovery in the book, *In an Instant: A Family's Journey of Love and Healing.*[56] The Woodruffs would go on to establish the Bob Woodruff Foundation, to assist our veterans and service members whose lives had been impacted by brain injuries.* As the newly appointed ABC news anchor, Woodruff was in Iraq in early 2006 covering the war by embedding with the troops when he suffered a severe brain injury. His vehicle directly encountered an improvised explosive device, (IED), which led to a severe brain injury, requiring emergent and life-saving neurosurgery. He was kept in a drug-induced coma for 36 days to reduce brain swelling, and his story of recovery is a testament to courage, not just for Mr. Woodruff, but for his wife and family.

Hope and encouragement are necessary to keep moving forward in recovery. Even in a coma it is not unusual for the comatose patient to have some sense of what is going on around the bedside. Whereas I had lost so much of my scientific skills after my injury, Woodruff lost much of his language skills. The irony that, for both of us, our injuries affected the brain hemisphere which we most relied on did not escape me.

In addition, upon reading Lee's book, I discovered that both he and I had that brain re-booting phenomenon, which came quite unexpectedly to me after weeks of my computer studies. Mr. Woodruff could not hide his injuries—he clearly had sustained

---

* The Bob Woodruff Foundation (http://bobwoodrufffoundation.org/) is a national nonprofit that helps ensure our nation's injured service members, veterans and their families return to a homefront ready to support them. Organizations like this one and The Resurrecting Lives Foundation (http://www.resurrectinglives.org/) offer resources to help those suffering from TBI to receive the most current rehabilitation options, and both are working to increase research and awareness of this ever increasing injury.

trauma to his brain as noted early on by the deformity in his skull. Unlike a patient with severe, visible injuries, those of us with mild TBI may expend energy toward convincing our colleagues and even our relatives that we have, in fact, suffered an injury at all. I wasn't exaggerating my disabilities. I wasn't right, and nothing I was doing was speeding the process for recovery, or so it seemed.

This brings about a very key point I've touched on before and will continue to speak to as I believe it is key to altering the outcome for TBI, especially mild TBI. It appears to me that one of the fundamental reasons for my and Woodruff's ultimate recovery was because we were blessed with an education and employment history which served as our basis for recovery. We both had access to experiences prior to our injuries that gave us the internal patterns for successful recoveries such as a history of intense education. After suffering our injuries, we both had access to advanced medical care and the financial support to focus our energy on recovery instead of merely on survival. How very different for our young military members; many of these young men and women volunteer to service directly after high school when the only knowledge stored on their hard drive is the knowledge of a young adult. This is a distinct disadvantage if you cannot recall old data, because you generally cannot lay down new data in the immediate post injury period. The brain recovery for new data retention will be different for everyone, but generally takes much longer than recalling stored data.

Due to the severity of his injuries, Woodruff attended multiple one-on-one rehabilitation sessions with various therapists: speech, occupational, physical. I, too, chose one-on-one therapy with me and my Mac (my Apple Macintosh computer, that is). No one could judge how impaired my speech or thought processes were, and no one would ever know just how debilitated and discouraged I felt on a daily basis.

How many of us are given the chance to make recovery their job? How many of our returning veterans are afforded the dignity they deserve both by the health care providers surrounding them and by the institutions built with the aim of serving them in return for their service to us? Given the rates of homelessness and poverty discussed previously in this book in relation to veterans returning to civilian life, I'd guess that it is very few who are afforded that opportunity, even with the VA's coordinated efforts to end homelessness among veterans. Given my experience as a volunteer within the VA hospital system, I can tell you anecdotally that many of those veterans I had diagnosed as having suffered a TBI nonetheless had to fight for a chance to receive benefits for that diagnosis. Eighty-five percent of the veterans I screened were diagnosed as having TBI and perhaps for that high number I was eventually removed from the volunteer physician roster, or so it appeared to me. A volunteer civilian physician was a new concept for the VA in 2009 but one that should be expanded, in my opinion. Sadly, I was one of the most trained TBI physicians at the time in a system that was already understaffed. Again, combining civilian and VA physicians with TBI experience is a win/win in the fight against the TBI epidemic. For all of our medical advances, without access to a timely diagnosis and rehabilitative support, recovery is greatly hampered.

While this is purely anecdotal on my part, I had found the ratio of spending about three hours of work on brain tasks that I was more easily able to handle to about one hour worth of specific work on what had become so very difficult for me to regain was a good strategy. The one hour of difficult tasks was very frustrating because so many days I simply got nowhere, just like in Woodruff's case, but I knew it was important to keep tweaking those circuits. Work and relax, not unlike a football player working hard on aerobic exercises one day and then strength the next—the cycle allowing for speedy, well-rounded improvements. That said, nothing comes quickly in recovering from a brain injury and that is one of the most difficult parts of being a caregiver—and I will echo that it is one of the most difficult parts of being a TBI sufferer.

One component of the brain's functional complexity is mirrored in the complexity of TBI received through differing forms of trauma. A newly released report by researchers funded through the Defense Health Program of the United States Department of Defense states that TBI from chronic blast exposure had a significantly different footprint of injury than TBI suffered by non-military members.[57] Furthermore, the report also highlighted that this level of specificity in brain injury research is so new that there are not yet any "evidence-based guidelines available for the definitive diagnosis or directed treatment of most blast-associated traumatic brain injuries, partly because the underlying pathology is unknown." In other words, going back to the beginning of this chapter, this is a reiteration of the concept that science doesn't trust what it doesn't know, and while it will take brave new research such as this to change what is or isn't known about the brain, your average physician still remains in the dark. Thankfully, non-profit organizations like the one I founded, Resurrecting Lives Foundation, and the very important One Mind for Research,[58] are combining resources of the military, the Veterans Administration, and the private sector to understand the brain. Co-founded by Garen and

Shari Staglin, and the Honorable Patrick Kennedy, with Retired General Peter Chiarelli as CEO, this non-profit shares the following organizational brief:

> *One Mind for Research is an independent, nonprofit organization committed to curing brain diseases and eliminating the stigma and discrimination they cause. In collaboration with partners in science, advocacy, and corporations, One Mind has developed an ambitious 10-year plan to radically accelerate the development of cures for brain diseases by changing the way scientists, health care professionals, NGOs, and government partners conduct research on brain disease and injury in order to accelerate delivery of improved diagnostics, treatments, and cures to patients.*[59]

As part of the chronic-blast research report mentioned above, the doctors included a series of images giving a clear indication of how different the brain of a blast-related TBI appears versus that of a TBI patient from another trauma. While this information does not yet provide a preferred treatment plan based on these individualistic traumas, it does help shine a light on yet another facet of how these injuries need to be considered when looking for an appropriate protocol path.

Dr. Lipton indicates that the damage present at the time of injury is also only one part of the overall damage that may ultimately occur. Currently there is no immediate at-the-time-of-concussion analysis that can be done to identify what has been damaged and what damage will evolve over time. In fact, most damage does not show up until days or weeks later because TBI is a progressive injury where axons may sustain damage and recover, or degenerate and even die, leading to loss of brain network function.

"One thing I can say is that the study we're involved in right now is large and complex, with hundreds of cases, and these are changes that are not manifest right away. If you look at what's gone on in the NFL, even cases of CTE are not due to a single head injury that happened at a specific point in time but to a lifetime of repeated injury. I think if we're fortunate enough to continue following these people over the next 5 to 10 years or more, we should have a much clearer understanding of the risk parameters; that's my optimistic side," Lipton said.

"What I hope is that people will continue to increase their understanding of the brain along with us, and understand it is both an incredibly complex and also delicate instrument to be handled gently," he continued. "Things that can cause serious stress on the brain need to be considered, like collision sports and military blasts, because prevention is always the better part of the cure."

Matt Bianco, an ex-defensive player and punt returner for the University of Dayton, said that while there was no single concussive event that led to him walking away from playing the sport, he had several injuries leading up to that life-changing decision.

"I'd had my first concussion in seventh grade after I knocked myself out snowboarding. I had full amnesia with that one. About three weeks after that my migraines began," Bianco said. "I started playing flag football at like five years old and as soon as I could play tackle ball I did. I probably had several other concussions but like a lot of guys just played through. My migraines always start with a visual impairment, like water covering your eyes making everything hazy until the vision blurs and the headache comes on."

During a punt return Bianco's junior year in an away game against Robert Morris University, he had a relatively routine helmet to helmet hit, striking the right side of his helmet and lower neck. Unfortunately, the result left him unconscious, and then he spent another 35-40 minutes in near blindness on the sidelines. This event essentially led to the conclusion of Bianco's football career.

As with so many young athletes, cumulative trauma may eventually lead to that one event that disrupts the brain pathways in such fashion as to render rehabilitation harder and longer than any previous event. When that happens, it is a difficult decision for the athlete who has to step away, especially after so many hours/weeks/ months/years of practice and conditioning to play the beloved sport of choice—whether it be football, soccer, hockey, or other contact sports. When the brain reacts in such a profound manner as Bianco describes above, it is often a life changing "incident." Every young athlete and military member must be aware of the second impact syndrome (SIS)[60] which occurs when a young brain swells rapidly and catastrophically after a person suffers a second concussion before the previous concussion is healed. The results are nearly uniformly fatal, and every high-risk sport and military operation must be monitored to avoid this catastrophic event because of the high mortality.

Beyond the story of Woodruff's recovery from his TBI and mine, I've found very minimal information regarding the lightning-strike moment of reboot. I don't believe this is due to a lack of experiences out there. More so, I see this missing evidence as part of the stigma surrounding our injured veterans and athletes.

These young men and women are already attempting to hide all they can from their families because, as Staff Sgt. Armstrong said, they feel in their core a need to protect their families from what happened in battle—and the battles they're fighting with themselves back at home. Another facet that is unfortunately problematic is that (not unlike many other internal diseases which have few to no external traumas) there are in fact some people who use the undiagnosed TBI or PTSD as a way of garnering attention for themselves, or attempting to take advantage of support systems put in place for those actually suffering. Cases like these, however few in number, only make it that much more difficult to find an appropriate path forward for the true heroes in need.

I never think my patients are crazy, because I know that they "are not out of their minds, they're out of their brains." In all fairness this is as much to do with who I am as it has to do with what I've been through myself. As mentioned in regard to Woodruff, and as I experienced, and as I've witnessed in other TBI sufferers—TBI patients are emotionally labile, hypervigilant, and they have what may seem like a short fuse. Realistically, TBI sufferers are living in a constant state of frustration with themselves, their brain-body connection, and the inability to communicate precisely what they are experiencing, and what they need, to those around them. The software and the hardware aren't working together properly, are constantly crashing, and need to be rebooted in order for some sense of consciousness to come forward and help produce a feeling of normality. No wonder we seem crazy to some people. Add to this the fact that the majority of our service personnel and first responders, who also suffer TBI as "work hazards," have always been the caretakers. This fact compounds the frustration. Police, firefighters, emergency response providers are often in harm's way, and suffer TBI as a result of their occupation. If these people become dependent and in need of care, a common response from their families is resentment, not just against the injury but against the injured themselves. Suffering a TBI can be a very lonely experience. Without caring and compassionate loved ones, it is no wonder there is a high rate of suicide amongst our injured heroes, those who volunteer to protect us here and abroad, who identify with being caregivers, first responders, or those gladiators on the playing field. All are left with few external resources when their internal resources fail.

Through this lens—one that lacks specific scientific information, lacks rehabilitation and recovery plans, and one that often lacks transparency with caregivers about what the TBI patient is suffering—it becomes apparent that experiencing a brain reboot and then immediately telling the world about it may not result in the resounding acceptance and exuberance you would hope for. As I mentioned previously, I felt the need to hide some amount of both my inabilities and of my recovery because I felt like those around me would question my reality even more than they already had.

My hope is that with more people sharing their stories as the Woodruffs have done, and as I am doing here, we will significantly increase awareness both in the medical community and in the general population, and that no one who has experienced a TBI is out-of-mind or crazy, but instead just temporarily out-of-their-brain.

In a *Scientific American* article titled "Time on the Brain: How You Are Always Living in the Past, and Other Quirks of Perception," George Musser wrote about the Foundational Questions Institute conference wherein they reported on how "our minds construct the past, present, and future, and sometimes get it badly wrong."[61]

The research, which included sufferers of TBI as well as a control group of healthy college students, suggested that memory is key to perceiving the future, and that the action of envisioning the future causes the same temporal patterns of activity as remembering the past. This changes, however, when we attempt to envision the future without any memory or using only factual information; that is when the brain seems unable to place ourselves into that future because we aren't able to use our past experience as the building blocks to construct that new future. Even in the best case scenario, throughout our life our brains do not store a "seamless narrative" but only "bits and pieces of what happened," which is why when we retrieve memories we are simultaneously using our intuition and creativity to construct (and possibly re-write) our past—the exact same sort of processing necessary to use stored information and experiences to predict a future event.

Anyone suffering a TBI that includes a loss of memory, large or small, is forced to live much more in the present than someone with an otherwise normal brain usually does. Consider how often in your day you spend thinking of either what happened before or what it is you're looking forward to, as opposed to focusing solely on your immediate task. When you've suffered a TBI you don't have the luxury of escape, and setting future goals becomes dramatically more difficult when you're unable to envision yourself in the future.

In recovery it is crucial then that for patient and caretaker alike, the present be recognized as the most important "time" as it can bring with it great gifts of light if only we're willing to accept them without trying to interpret those points of light through what came before, or subject them to a future that can't be clearly seen and may never come to be.

CHAPTER NINE

THE CITY LIGHTS

Driving a car in traffic when you are only comfortable, and really only able, to make right turns is at best a time-consuming proposition and to be more frank, a flat-out annoyance. The right hand turn is more comfortable for a good reason here in the United States—you only need to judge the arc of the turn and avoid pedestrians who are much slower moving than other vehicles.

I was not at all what you might call healed at this point, about six months into my recovery, but I would surmise that about 65 percent of my knowledge had been restored, or at least I knew the resource to retrieve it, so I decided I would press on with my rehabilitation efforts. For the following year I could only make right hand turns because the extremely complex thought process necessary to make a left hand turn still escaped me. Left hand turns represent the majority of fatal crashes for the elderly in the US because of the need for your brain to process all of the spatial details of the turn itself, which may or may not include an additional lane of traffic, as well as the speed of any oncoming traffic and the timing necessary for successfully executing the turn. I was cognizant of my inability to negotiate these turns, and therefore willing to take the extra time required to drive with only right turn capabilities. After all, unless I could get to my patients, I could not continue my own rehab. Being a caregiver, again, instead of a care taker was key for my recovery, as it is for our service personnel. Like so many of them, I had always relied on myself, and was very aware that others relied on me as well.

This driving freedom buoyed my enthusiasm as I continued working my rehab "three hour to one" strategy. I stepped up the content to include more complex calculations, taking on some Shakespeare instead of just "see Spot run" books. Altogether these steps renewed my belief that I was getting better, even if it remained a series of starts and stops, low periods and then sudden leaps as the circuits reconnected and the lights came on.

My days were getting more normal at this point as well. I was still sleeping longer than I ever had in my life, getting to sleep about 10 p.m. and up around 8 a.m. Instead of seeing patients once an hour I was back to my 30-minute appointments and, of course, had figured out my right-hand-turn-only route to work so that I could drive myself, which was no small victory in my mind. In fact, it wasn't until a year after my accident that I began trusting myself to make left hand turns when driving.

Even with a growing normality (or at least regularity) to my life I was completely terrified by the prospect of going off the amantadine that had helped to reboot my brain and bring back my speech, vision, and other faculties. I called my physician and asked how much longer I should continue taking the medication. He confirmed my concern by saying he felt it was time to get off the amantadine, that it likely had done all that it could. Because of my fear and dread over the potential for reverting back to my pre-medicated self I chose to wean my way off the drug. I had been on 100 mg every six hours through this point so I dropped that down to every eight hours over the next couple of weeks. Thankfully there was no change and I felt comfortable spending a couple more weeks at one dose every 12 hours before switching to one per day and then, a month or so later, going amantadine-free.

Like an addict who isn't yet convinced they're done with their drug, I kept a stash of amantadine hidden away for a long time, maybe another year or so, just in case I needed it. Thankfully I never did. The thing is, TBI patients rehabilitating themselves must be willing (and allowed) to make small changes over time, weaning instead of white knuckling, because even a healthy brain can only filter so much noise, but a brain in recovery has a much lower tolerance for change—for separating the important signals from the noisy ones.

A surprising tidbit is that the majority of what the brain does when engaging with your sensory organs is to filter out activity and information, as opposed to trying to gather additional information, allowing only what is necessary to be processed to make it that far in. I still wasn't filtering out enough information at this point so I avoided anything I could that might overstimulate my brain.

A classic hallmark primarily connected with the PTSD diagnosis that we are now understanding is equally true of TBI is a perceived avoidance of people, particularly large crowds. The myth we must dispel is that this is purely an emotional response that can be medicated away with anxiety drugs or other psychotropic medications. These medications may alleviate some symptoms of anxiety but do not help heal the brain processes that are responsible for filtering, and may leave patients even more vulnerable by increasing stress on the very brain functions that need to heal.

For over a year I avoided going into any large stores, the mall, stadiums—pretty much anywhere that I would be subject to large crowds, intense lighting, or loud noise. During that time, I even did all of my grocery shopping at the United Dairy Farmers near my house—a small Ohio-based chain of corner convenience stores. This meant that my diet consisted primarily of peanut butter and jelly sandwiches, cheese sandwiches, cereal, and ice cream. I'd like to admit that I have anecdotal evidence that my dietary changes influenced my recovery, but in reality, I'd have a hard time suggesting that this part of my rehabilitation was the best it could be.

Given that I had entered this period of cautious optimism that I would in fact get back to some semblance of my old self, I was leaning heavily on the side of caution. I began exercising again with more regularity as I had done prior to my injury, but with more boundaries. Instead of an every-single-day regimen I relegated myself to about 20 minutes a day three times a week on the treadmill. Weight training brought on headaches, so I backed off on that. I was trying not to get another TBI. As we now know, once you have suffered a TBI you are three times more likely to suffer another TBI, often from losing control of your body or your balance and falling.

Interestingly, in a study titled "Pre-existing Health Conditions and Repeat Traumatic Brain Injury" by Lee L. Saunders, PhD, and others, the researchers discovered that besides the more seemingly obvious conditions that would lead to repeat TBI, such as alcohol and drug abuse or high-risk job and athletic activities, the lack of insurance and lower socioeconomic status also brought about a significant increase.[62]

"We found that insurance status was significantly associated with repeat TBI, with persons who had Medicaid or who were uninsured having a higher rate of repeat TBI than persons with commercial insurance," the study states. As we know, lack of affordable healthcare in the United States remains a significant issue, even under the Affordable Care Act, and as we've discussed earlier in the book there have been significant challenges on behalf of the VA hospitals to provide TBI care to our veterans. In addition to insurance and coverage, of course, the spatial, visual, and balance difficulties surrounding a TBI make a second injury more probable, especially early on in the healing process.

In early 2008 I began my stint volunteering with a VA hospital here in Ohio until I was quite abruptly asked to end my tour of duty there on March 17, 2009. I had been providing second-level screening for potential TBI sufferers, most of whom had originally been told their issues were related to PTSD, which the VA has consistently treated as more of an emotional disorder instead of as an actual brain injury. Once again this proves that the medical system does not like what it can't explain—in this case treating a brain injury like a "mental" illness with anti-depressants and other psychotropic medications. We are on the verge of identifying the brain processes: the chemical and chemical receptor issues surrounding all of brain health, including what we now label as a "mental" disorder. Brain research with new neuroradiological techniques has increased our knowledge dramatically in the last decade. Yet, as stated previously in this book, it is estimated that only

8-10 percent of all health care professionals actually treat traumatic brain injuries. As noted earlier, most of these are treatments for moderate to severe injuries, not those classified as "mild."

I had been inspired to volunteer at the VA by the death of a young man I'd been familiar with, Sgt. Zachary Wade McBride (killed in action, Sinsil, Iraq, at 20 years old). The mantra of honoring our fallen by caring for their brothers and sisters who return from action became my call to action. From my very first patient who claimed to have been diagnosed with PTSD, I began uncovering more and more of these veterans who may have also had PTSD, but likewise had suffered a TBI. Yet, they were not receiving the appropriate care from the VA clinics for the diagnosis. What we know is that our heroes are out of their brains, they are not crazy, and are not out of their minds.

Post traumatic *brain* disorder is a real thing as I've stated before in this book, and has a co-morbidity with TBI; however, it is a chemical assault on the brain causing a continuous loop of brain activity hard to break out of. Rebalancing this chemical change is a game of chess, the same as finding ways to reconnect broken neural pathways associated with the physical assault on the brain that is a traumatic brain injury. In chess though, the way you win is not to just randomly throw all your pawns into the scrum and hope they'll overwhelm the enemy; instead, a methodical strategy must be laid out, followed up with tactical decisions in support of that strategy.

In a world of ever-tightening budgets for public institutions such as the VA, there has been a lack of will to invest in the metaphorical chess players and the potentially time-consuming treatment plans required to win. For my part, I had become a liability to the VA, correctly diagnosing TBI patients when the VA found it more efficient to label them with a PTSD diagnosis. After all, the VA had defined PTSD in the Vietnam Era, long before we acquired the capability of imaging the brain. It was time to make a change, and the swifter the change was made, the greater the opportunity to correctly diagnose and treat the brain.

Journalist Daniel Zwerdling (NPR and ProPublica) reported in June 2010 that back in 2007, prior to my joining the VA, the military had come under enormous pressure to "fix problems in diagnosing and treating brain injuries. Yet despite the hundreds of millions of dollars pumped into the effort since then, critical parts of this promise remain unfulfilled."[63] Among the findings Zwerdling reported were:

- "From the battlefield to the homefront, the military's doctors and screening systems routinely miss brain trauma in soldiers. One of the military tests fails to catch as many as 40 percent of concussions, a recent unpublished study concluded. A second exam, on which the Pentagon has spent millions, yields results that top medical officials call about as reliable as a coin flip.

- "Even when military doctors diagnose head injuries, that information often doesn't make it into soldiers' permanent medical files. Handheld medical devices designed to transmit data have failed in the austere terrain of the war zones. Paper records from Iraq and Afghanistan have been lost, burned or abandoned in warehouses, officials say, when no one knew where to ship them.

- "Without diagnosis and official documentation, soldiers with head wounds have had to battle for appropriate treatment. Some received psychotropic drugs instead of rehabilitative therapy that could help retrain their brains. Others say they have received no treatment at all, or have been branded as malingerers."

As Staff Sgt. Armstrong explained to me when we first met, he was having a terrible time getting the VA to do anything but prescribe him a variety of anti-depressant and pain killing medications, none of which were really helping beyond providing some feeling of numbness to the chaos going on inside his head. During an interview with him in 2016 for this book, he reiterated the fact that he still struggles to receive treatment and support from the VA. Research doctor Jeffrey Greenberg, PhD., likens what is occurring in the VA and other clinics serving our military with the famous Bernard Baruch statement, "If all you have is a hammer, everything looks like a nail." It often takes years to change accepted practices.

Greenberg questions the common response of diagnosing PTSD when it is very possible something else is going on, such as TBI, actual depression, or another health issue altogether, such as failure of the pituitary gland, the main controller of hormonal activity in the body. He is particularly interested in this science of problem solving, and you could definitely call him a chess player in this realm.

"The science of problem solving tells us that to solve a problem, we must first understand it. This requires a global or holistic perspective on the total health of our returned service members. We remain challenged to understand the complex relationships between head injuries and psychological health problems. Assessment, diagnostics, and treatment of these complex problems are difficult," Greenberg said. "We are uncertain what types of treatment wounded warriors are receiving. Are they evidence-based treatments, and are they delivered with fidelity? Are the diagnostics accurate?"[64]

His assertion that I want to echo is that if the application of an appropriate treatment is not made then the result is "that the treatment will fail the individual, not the other way around." We cannot continue to fail our injured veterans who have fought so valiantly for us, nor our athletes who have captivated us with their athleticism.

As we've now discussed repeatedly, there are no fully vetted protocols in place for diagnosis and treatment of these brain issues at this time—and anything that has been introduced is still very much in uncharted territory. What I hope you, our fearless and faithful reader, will consider as we bring this text towards its end is helping to ask our representatives and decision makers to fully fund the research necessary to finally win this game of chess and to put practical and effective protocols in place for not just the current generation, but future generations as well.

We need to bring light to every veteran suffering in every city across this country. I know that rehabilitation and recovery are possible. I join many others as living proof of that. However, knowing that it is possible is only the first step along a long and sometimes dark road of discovery. The research in the private sector has provided signs along the way, revealing some positive outcomes. Primarily, those outcomes are coming from: cognitive processing and rehabilitative therapy, hyperbaric oxygen, transcendental meditation, exercise (particularly yoga), physical therapy, speech therapy, occupational therapy, and creativity-oriented therapies such as music and art. Positive outcomes are also resulting from use of medications such as modafinil and amantadine, including some other stimulants that are closely monitored and carefully adjusted to provide primarily short-term stabilization and recovery gains. Pituitary replacement is key if this gland has failed as a result of blast forces. Brief periods of anti-depressants and other medications may also be appropriate in some cases, but require close assessment; psychotropic medicines should not be used since this research has already found these to be harmful to TBI sufferers as they may be merely masking underlying issues or even exacerbating them. Finally, as discussed earlier, even medical marijuana may be helpful, but given the inconsistent laws currently in place it has been difficult to prove this without objective research.

Ultimately it will take objective research to either prove or dispel all these treatments. Otherwise the medical community will be unwilling to embrace them. For many practitioners, this may be a hindrance to treating TBI patients at all.

Thanks to the direction of the VA Secretary, David Shulkin, MD, and his predecessor, Robert McDonald, strides to deliver specialty care are being made through the Choice Act, allowing veterans to seek specialty care for brain injuries. Although the system is still working out the processing difficulties of scheduling and reimbursement for specialists, the 2014 VACAA (Veterans Access, Choices, and Accountability Act) remains a bipartisan response aimed at solving access to specialists issues for our veterans. It is a start.

CHAPTER TEN

A NEW BALANCE LIGHTING THE WAY

While recovering from a TBI, it is difficult to become introspective. You spend so much time and energy just getting through the day's reduced activities that there is no energy left for reflection. Nearly a decade later in my recovery I finally had the room for reflection and realized that my recovery was also my boot-camp for my work with veterans struggling with TBI.

Like the injury itself, the realization dawned on me rather abruptly while I was evaluating my first veteran at a VA outpatient clinic in Ohio. After requiring the young soldier to complete a computer-based, multiple-screen evaluation, I chose to take it too, out of curiosity. To my surprise, according to the VA program, I was diagnosed as having PTSD, not TBI. I related to my patient in that I shared many of his symptoms of hypervigilance, avoidance of crowds, lowered frustration threshold, and decreased tolerance to noise and light. I then explained that I sustained my injury while putting up Christmas lights, and his immediate reaction ultimately changed my life. I'll never forget it.

No sooner had I muttered the words, "decorating the house for Christmas," he seized my wrist, looked me squarely in the eye and proclaimed, "So what you mean, Doc, is that I'm not crazy!"

Wow! That hit me like a Humvee. Here, staring at my face for a reaction, was a young soldier who had survived serving two tours of duty in Iraq and eight IED explosions asking me—no, begging me to legitimize his condition as a physical injury, not a mental illness. In that moment, I asked myself two questions: (1) just how many thousands of patients with brain injuries think they're crazy? And (2) how can we, as physicians, correct this stigma of hopelessness?

A year later I would begin to answer those questions when I read the RAND Report, brilliantly researched and championed by study co-director Terri Tanielian, which explained that 25 percent of our veterans from Iraq and Afghanistan suffer from TBI.[65] The intel from Rand set me on a mission to film the documentary, *Operation Resurrection*,[66] to engage civilian resources as a way of bringing attention to the problem and hopefully creating awareness in the public sector. The military represents 1 percent of the US population, whereas the civilian world represents the remaining 99 percent of the population and resources. We need to assist the Department of Defense and the Veterans Administration in collaborations for providing the best health care, education, and employment opportunities to these injured veterans and their families.

In pursuit of my mission, I learned about the efforts of Army Brigadier General Loree Sutton, MD, a psychiatrist who served in a visionary leadership role, lighting the way forward to bring our injured heroes the sort of advanced diagnostic and rehabilitation services they deserved. Brig. Gen. Sutton served as founding director for the Defense Centers of Excellence for Psychological Health and Traumatic Brain Injury, DCoE, a congressionally-mandated center created to respond to the growing needs of our military members with TBI. The DCoE oversees three centers, each contributing to the fields of psychological health and traumatic brain injury. The centers include: Defense and Veterans Brain Injury Center (DVBIC), the Deployment Health Clinical Center (DHCC), and the National Center of Telehealth and Technology (T2).

In addition to the DCoE created by Congress, there is a network of rehabilitation centers built using $65 million in private donations from the public. The Intrepid Fallen Heroes Fund (IFHF), created by the Fisher family, led the fundraising effort. The IFHF has funded nine other centers since this one, called Intrepid Spirit centers, which are located on major military bases throughout the country and were constructed under the guidance of Arnie Fisher, a New York real estate investor, philanthropist, and patriot. These collaborative efforts by Fisher, the Fisher Foundation, and the DoD represent how combining civilian and military resources solves problems. Together, we can alleviate the TBI epidemic.

As both a physician and a military leader, Brig. Gen. Sutton had a clear understanding for the need to implement the DCoE with a focus on TBI and psychological health issues associated with military service. Brig. Gen. Sutton was also instrumental in coordinating efforts between Dr. Michael Lipton and my work with veterans, bringing additional research with neuroradiology techniques that would expand the conversation about TBI diagnosis and treatment, while proving that collaboration with the civilian health care resources is not only necessary but achievable. I was fortunate, and more importantly, our returning military with TBI were fortunate, to partake in research with Dr. Lipton, approved by Brig. Gen. Sutton, to link the effects of IED blasts on the brain. Through the use of newer radiographic techniques, especially diffusion tensor imaging, DTI, the link between blast and brain injury was confirmed, a discovery which has been reconfirmed in further studies by Dr. David Brody, MD, PhD at Washington University in St. Louis. Recently she was appointed by New York Mayor Bill De Blasio in the leadership role in the city's Department of Veterans' Services, where she continues to champion successful re-entry into the civilian world, including her participation in the development of a community-oriented program called Life in the New Normal, aimed at helping to build strong, emotionally healthy military families who have to deal with a loved one suffering the effects of TBI or psychological (among other) issues.

Leadership like that being offered by Brig. Gen (Ret.) Sutton has been slowly gaining traction and depth over the past year. While the NFL settled a $900 million lawsuit with about 5,000 former players in 2013, it wasn't until February 2016 that Jeff Miller, the NFL's senior vice president for health and safety, acknowledged the link between football-related head trauma and CTE.[67] This admission opened that settlement up to appeal, part of the lawsuit that Jonathan Wells is part of, because the settlement originally had been made under the exclusion of future cases of CTE, as well as not covering known co-morbid issues such as depression and mood disorders. Prior to Miller making the surprise announcement, the NFL leadership had continued to claim that there was no definite link between sports-related head trauma and CTE or any other TBI symptoms.

Paraphrasing the old 12-step program cliché, "Admitting we have a problem is the first step." Admission of a problem has seemingly been the popular notion among athletic organizations and government officials over the past year—but that must be translated into action. Grassroots non-profit organizations such as the Resurrecting Lives Foundation are helping to work directly with the DoD to coordinate the health care and employment opportunities of military members as they reintegrate as veterans. We are partnering with other private and public organizations to continue shining a light on this issue.

For myself, I've always found activities such as hiking and dancing to be therapeutic. I remember when I first felt comfortable enough to lace on my favorite New Balance running shoes and get back to my treadmill; there was an irony to the event because looking at those shoes I realized I too had arrived at a "new balance" in my own life. Even though I'd lost my nearly photographic memory, and my ability to understand geography and location had mostly disappeared, I knew I could power walk in the safety of my own home thanks to my trusty trainers and my treadmill. Through that exercise, I cleared my brain of all other distractions and began to feel comfortable in my own personal "new normal," which brought about this new balance to my life.

All that I had lost, that I've talked over throughout this book—my very deep skillset for science and mathematics, my ability to quickly learn new subject matter and names, my ability to multitask—I know now that it was not all lost without also contributing some gifts. Prior to my TBI I was a scientist, a workaholic and an all-business left-brained person. After my TBI and recovery I found my right brain significantly improved, providing me with a desire to be creative that I'd never felt before. Combine this creative drive with a loss of my inhibition to more publicly take on perceived injustices and before I knew it, I was heading up the production of a documentary film, *Operation Resurrection*, posing the questions, "Why don't the VA, the DoD, and other available resources work together for the health care, employment and education of our all-voluntary military members when they discharge from service?" I'd never had the motivation or drive to write anything more than what a patient chart or prescription pad required of me, but I soon found myself writing poetry, music, lyrics, and now even this book. Fortunately, over time much of my scientific and mathematical skills have come back; but I know now how much more color to life there can be by having had my right brain elevated beyond my left. Before my TBI I never would've had the audacity to become a mirror for the DoD and the VA to suggest the corrective activities for our veterans—but here I am today attempting to be and do just that.

Staff Sgt. Armstrong and other veterans who I've had the honor of working with have also taken lead roles in retelling their denials by the VA for TBI benefits, likened to the denial by tobacco companies in regard to lung cancer. These military members that fought so bravely for the United States now are not just leading the fight for their own care, but advocating and fighting for all of their brothers and sisters in arms. They are testifying before Congress, helping each other with navigating the VA bureaucracy, and attending fundraising events to help bring in research monies and broaden the base of advocates who hope that one day our government and institutions choose to take as good care of these heroes as our heroes have taken of all of us.

I prefer not to come across as negative, or angry, over the way things have played out, but there are times I have difficulty expressing myself in any other way because one significant trademark of TBI is a quickening of temper, and a lessening of patience. This trait doesn't have to be all negative though, and I think this is an important consideration for both those suffering TBI and their caregivers. I have always had a tendency toward hypomania—the need to be constantly in motion, tackling new challenges and following my curiosity to conclusion. While impatience and anger can cause a sort of blindness, they both tend to boost energy; so redirecting that energy, like what I've done and what Staff Sgt. Armstrong has done, just might be what we all need to win this war.

Not long after production of the documentary film *Operation Resurrection* had gotten underway, the light that the filmmakers and I were shining on the VA bureaucracy's inability to deal with our growing number of injured military led to one of the VA regional directors attempting to stall our work. Were it not for my upbringing and my new found assertiveness in this realm, I don't think the documentary would've been completed—nor this book ever started.

By fall 2012, our attempts to make public records requests and to get interviews with VA staff members in charge of both the care and the determination of eligibility for care felt like a battle we were losing at times—but like any military member knows, you don't often have the luxury of picking your battle, those are usually chosen for you by fate or function.

I think often about the military creed of "protecting our own," and it kept in sight for me all who had gone into battle and protected us without hesitation. I can no longer hesitate in this fight for protecting these heroes I now see as my "own" as well—brave men and women I'd come to identify with so clearly due to our shared affliction, and our shared patriotism, and our shared desire for justice and doing what is morally and ethically right.

Football legend Harry Carson and I shared the stage at an Ohio Osteopathic Physician education event at the NFL Football Hall of Fame in 2015. Carson is not merely a hero of mine, in football and in life, but also a mentor, who leads the battle to fight for the care of NFL athletes, and really, for anyone who is suffering from TBI—even me. In October 2015, the NFL had not yet turned the corner on accepting that football-related TBI may be connected to the increasing number of current and ex-NFL players suffering from brain disorders and committing suicide. It was so interesting to me that this medical conference was held at the Canton Football Hall of Fame, but not sanctioned by the institution, nor the NFL. Still, it was an amazing opportunity to address these issues—"TBI from the Battlefield to the Playing Field"—to such an interested audience.

The reason for stating all of this may have, at one point in my life, been specifically to draw attention to put pressure on the institutions unwilling to consider the research. However, thanks to those people who I've mentioned previously standing up over recent years we are now at a point where we see how their fighting spirit, our fighting spirit, has produced results. We have too much on the line not to keep fighting, and recent events such as the expansion of the Intrepid Centers for our military members are clear victories. The NFL announcement by the senior vice-president of health and safety, Jeff Miller, shows that we are winning battles and headed toward winning the war. Just two years earlier, in 2013, five young veterans accompanied me to Capitol Hill where we were even able to screen our documentary to provide testimony to over 150 staff members of the US House and Senate interested in veterans' health, education, and employment.

Around the time of our documentary being released, Army Dr. Col. Geoffrey Ling, a program manager (now retired) at the Defense Advanced Research Projects Agency (DARPA), announced in an address to medical care providers at NICoE, that the "Gray Team" he served on (a group of five combat doctors) were pursuing mandatory TBI screening that at the time was dubbed MACE (Military Acute Concussion Evaluation).[68] Army Col. Dr. Christian Macedonia had been charged with creating and leading the Gray Team after suffering a TBI of his own during a mortar attack on his combat zone medical center. The attack had left him unable to remember what had happened the day before. Realizing how few soldiers were even being screened for TBI post-IED and other concussive battlefield explosions, Macedonia knew he had to take the lead on changing the situation.

"Quite simply, the Gray Team was there to establish ground truth with respect to traumatic brain injury," Macedonia said in an interview for NPR.[69] "The organized military medical system was still trying to hold back the ocean and say: No big deal, most of these injuries are psychiatric and our job is basically to provide counseling centers and get these people over the shock of being at war."

Citing the same bureaucratic concerns that I had faced, Macedonia said, "I can't tell you the number of times I walked out of rooms just being sorely disappointed at people who knew what the right thing to do was but chose to look the other way." Reports by Gray Team members documented by the military and in interviews with NPR, *The New York Times*, and *Nature International Weekly Journal of Science* suggested at the time that only about 10 percent of wounded combat soldiers were being assessed.

Fortunately, as of the writing of this book, the NFL, FIFA, and several other major sporting governance bodies recognize TBI for the danger that it is and are working on ways to better inform and protect athletes participating in those events.

Luke Johnson, former quarterback for the University of Dayton Flyers stated, "I'd be hard pressed to find anyone I know from playing football as a kid, in high school, or at the college level who hasn't had a concussion. I just think the big problem is they go undiagnosed," Johnson said. "Like with Matt [Bianco]—we'd go out on a Saturday night and it was just clear to me how tired he was from taking so many hits, and how you'd be in like a fog for a couple days. Part of going undiagnosed is the culture, you're making sacrifices for your brothers on the field and a winning season. No one wants to use the "concussion" word on the sidelines.

"I don't think this is the exception but the general rule. When you consider that Matt and I both knew we weren't going on to the NFL but kept playing because we thought we had to, well, then put that into perspective of the guys whose only real hope for making it in life is getting to the NFL or some other pro league, there's just a lot on the line for those guys and the people they take care of," Johnson said.

Bianco agreed and added how this is multiplied in regard to our heroes in the military.

"In a sport you're not depending on each other for your life, but this is even more prominent in the military where you're not just a liability to yourself or a game, but for your life," Bianco said.

Also as of the writing of this book, the VA has significantly increased their resources focused on the study of TBI and PTSD-related issues, including running several internal treatment studies aimed at moving the organization's strategy of care forward. The CogSMART program discussed earlier was studied by the VA for implementation beginning in mid-2014, and a new, 10-year study called MIND (Markers for the Identification, Norming, and Differentiation of TBI and PTSD) is now underway. Both the DoD and VA have responded rather quickly, considering the extent of that bureaucracy and the scope of the TBI issue.

Members of the Gray Team continue to shine light on these issues even after moving on from their military service. Team member and Harvard researcher Dr. Parker (mentioned earlier in the book) had originally been a cellular biologist researcher focused on heart-related issues and didn't get interested in TBI until a close friend of his that he'd served with in the army gave him a call. Parker said that after reconnecting it was clear something wasn't right with his friend, and what was going on seemed like something more than the PTSD he'd been diagnosed with; it seemed like something was wrong with his brain.

Parker already had a long list of credits to his name at this point including publications like the *Journal of Applied Physiology*, mostly related to how seemingly minor shockwaves hitting the cells in the heart can create an immediate, and possibly fatal, heart attack.[70] The damage, although life-threatening, in and of itself doesn't leave any significant markers at the cellular level. His research on behalf of his friend's TBI led to the discovery of a neural protein connector called integrin, which triggers chemical pathways for interactions between brain cells. According to Parker, in much the same way that the heart can stop from a shockwave with little or no cellular damage, it appears the brain's integrin connections (also known as bridges) can be broken or altered by a blast shockwave leaving behind a mostly invisible, but very real, physical brain injury.[71]

This research on proteins unfortunately has yet to catch the eye of the pharmaceutical industry, a point Parker has been quick to point out in several interviews because he believes their participation is crucial to finding a drug that will actually heal these integrin connections. For his part, he and his lab are trying to identify more specific proteins for pharmaceutical companies to target, hoping that by doing some of the difficult and costly puzzling out of this information they might bring about greater interest in the field.

About what he could ultimately consider success in this battle, Parker told NPR, "Success is that a quarterback doesn't suffer from dementia after being sacked. Success is that brain injury is no longer the leading cause of death of children. Success is a war fighter gets blown up in some Third World rat-hole somewhere and he can still count his change at Burger King afterwards."

"It's a very personal issue for us. This is not an occupation. This is an obsession."

Of course we are optimistic about these more recent, progressive steps by our military, our government, our athletic organizations, and our civilian researchers, but these changes will only continue to improve and become permanent if we all light the way and embrace this need, making that support known loud and clear. Echoing Parker, I agree that this is a very personal issue and we must all be obsessive about it if we're going to win the war against TBI.

Only then will all of our suffering TBI patients find the light and reclaim their personal new balance.

CHAPTER ELEVEN

SHARING THE LIGHT

Since 2008, when my tour of duty began into the world of TBI assessment amongst our veterans, I stopped all other interests I had and found myself obsessing over this epidemic. My only mission was to find a way to improve the military separation process for our service personnel and their families, providing a sound plan upon military separation. We, as a nation, need to do this in a way our veterans can not only adjust to civilian life, but thrive as a result of their voluntary service to our nation.

As of right now, we have nearly one million patients willing to be studied and diagnosed with either PTSD (a likely diagnosis they've already received, whether it was accurate or not) or as having suffered a TBI. Information sharing would include the Pentagon opening its data about rates of TBI and PTSD. Spokespersons have voiced concern that sharing any data associated with battlefield injuries and deaths may put active duty soldiers at risk. Without that data, however, we continue to put the injured who may or may not have a proper diagnosis at risk. The difference between a PTSD diagnosis and a TBI diagnosis is the difference of about $2,500 in benefits to cover the first year of treatment for PTSD with medications, versus $25,000 to cover the first-year treatment for TBI with therapies including speech, physical, and occupational. Once we accurately provide a diagnosis, the real work towards recovery and reintegration into civilian society can occur, but not before then.

Sharing this mission is going to take an army of interested individuals and organizations collaborating, including looking for new ways to provide a smooth and seamless transition of medical records and patient information between the VA and other public clinics, as well as private health care providers. Currently, the hand-off of this information requires significant effort on the part of the patient or their caregivers.

"I can't begin to tell you how many times I've had to request paperwork from the VA or the Army in an attempt to get the records I need to get basic doctor appointments," Staff Sgt. Armstrong told me. "Once I had them, I felt like I had to guard them with my life because I didn't want to try and get them again, it really sucks."

To this end, without a genuinely cooperative effort between the Department of Defense, the VA, and our civilian health care system, advocating for open and unbiased research into TBI diagnosis and treatment will be next to impossible. We do have advocates, however, including Gen. (Ret.) Peter Chiarelli, who heads up Patrick Kennedy's One Mind for Research Foundation, as well as former VA Secretary Bob McDonald, who attempted to ease the bureaucratic blockade through the Choice Act. Opening up partnerships and intelligence sharing between public and private sectors could create incredible opportunities for joint research with financially stable organizations such as the NFL. My hope is that we find a way to unite our efforts to protect and care for one of our nation's greatest resources: our volunteer military members and their families.

Reading back over what I've written leads me to keep one of my mantras at the forefront of my mind: "Try to be patient." Do not give up and yet, do not fool yourself into thinking that you will be the same after the journey. This statement is as true for me individually, as a person who has suffered and rehabilitated from a TBI, as well as for the various organizations that I expect will find a way to partner together and solve this problem, even if I must drag them one by one to the table. Being patient does not mean you can't also be tenacious. After my accident, I knew I didn't want to be where I was. I also knew, however, that as a scientist I would learn something from the experience which would help me to assist others. If I hadn't believed that, I would never have worked so hard to find the light outside the darkness that I'd been plunged into.

Many things blessed me during my recovery. I did not have a team of caregivers, as that has never been my fate. Instead, I was blessed because I had a decent brain before the injury, at least in my estimation, and the recovery kept me able to serve others, to continue to learn from my patients. Without being of service to others, I would've felt I had little purpose in my life. We are here to help each other by using whatever talents we have been given. If I ever remember one Bible story well, it's the one about the talents bestowed upon us. The first time I felt I really understood this passage was during Sunday school, at about five years old: "To those whom God has given much, much is expected."

I live by that rule because it makes so much sense to me, especially on the heels of suffering a TBI that could have rendered me utterly incapable of even taking care of myself. Every experience I have now I try to use to make the world a gentler place for someone else. It sounds cliché, I know, but it's how I feel. Without feeling this way, the whole TBI would have been a waste of my efforts and my talents.

Throughout the book, and in person, I often speak about my *former brain*, which was much sharper than my current brain. Although it may have been much more intelligent, it was also much less creative and, I must say, much more censored. When I spoke to the Army Medical Corps at Ft. Sam Houston, for instance, I commented that my former brain, my "Catholic school-trained brain," would have never been comfortable on stage speaking to 400 service members in the auditorium, not to mention another 1,000 via a nationwide video conference regarding the need to change their belief system. This new brain of mine had no difficulty reflecting that light of what it means to navigate a broken system with a TBI. I found myself speaking from the truth that only comes when you have overcome something so difficult, when you now can climb down into that hole your friend is trapped in because, now, you know the way out. There is no way I would be doing this for myself, but I'm so thankful to have this mission to keep me from remaining introverted and ultimately alone. To say that my life has changed would be a complete understatement; it has been revolutionized. The irony of God's plan is that he chose an introverted pacifist to be the champion for warriors. Who would have planned that one?

While I recognize that in myself, and even in some of my heroes who have served as warriors themselves, so many of us involved in this fight also came from blue-collar backgrounds where we learned early on that we all had to stick together and support the underdog if we were going to get by. I grew up in Youngstown, Ohio, also deemed "murder town USA" when I was a kid. We rooted for the Browns and the Indians; we were the undisputed champions of the underdogs. So, taking this mission on was ultimately something I had been born into without realizing it. Or, maybe a better way of saying this is that it took losing my brain to find my mission.

No one is more deserving of our expert medical care than our veterans who have sustained injuries in defense of our nation. Whether it be in boot camp or combat, they provide our protection, and we should honor their commitment to us by committing to their healing upon their return to the civilian world. Veterans returning from OIF and OEF who had never been given the opportunity to receive a proper diagnosis or treatment are just as victimized of injustice as our Vietnam Era veterans who suffered contact with Agent Orange but never received any treatment. We cannot, as a nation, continue to cover up these purportedly "invisible" wounds of war. We either go all in as a nation, or we stop going to war at all. Like many people looking to change the world, it is my sense of justice that ultimately drives me to shine a spotlight on what our military members, veterans, and their families are experiencing.

Thankfully, I'm not alone in this battle. Besides the people I've mentioned by name or by organization, the board members of the Resurrecting Lives Foundation are engaged in multiple presentations every year, as am I, resulting in outreach at over 100 different events related to the issue of TBI and PTSD. The board as a whole attempts to exponentially increase our reach by taking to social media and inviting every vet we've had contact with to do the same, networking further through their family and friends as a pay-it-forward service.

Bianco and his fellow teammate, former University of Dayton quarterback Luke Johnson, joined this work through the non-profit Resurrecting Lives Foundation partnership with Cardinal Health in hopes of positively impacting other veterans who may be at risk of TBI, or in recovery from one.

"I had some time to think about advice I received while making my decision to quit playing football," Bianco said during our last meeting. "It came from my coaches and personal doctor, and it was whether I could continue to play and not be hesitant. The guy who is hesitant is typically the one who gets hurt. If I were ever to be able to play the game and continue to play at the level I wanted, I knew I was going to be hesitant about taking more hits, and therefore decided against returning to the sport.

"It was more than just realizing where you stand; it was also about getting second and third opinions. I went to about four doctors and just talked about my injuries. I also saw a psychologist, to help me understand if there may be some mental health issues at hand. But I had the fortune of all of these resources, and many athletes do not, so I think the best advice is about at the very least understanding whether or not you can continue to play at such an intense level and do so safely," Bianco said.

Through the generous public donations and the incredible support of AMVETS Post #26 in Mansfield, Ohio, Resurrecting Lives Foundation was able to fund research at Albert Einstein College of Medicine, where Dr. Lipton proved the anatomy of TBI associated with blast injuries at a time that the VA and DoD insisted that the previous research of the issue was equivocal. Dr. Lipton's findings on our pilot research assisted other leading researchers, including Dr. David Brody, to test our findings on a much larger scale. Brody completed a second study where he managed to further Lipton's research while also verifying the accuracy of Lipton's discoveries.[72]

Our biggest roadblock at this point seems to be the bean counters—"How much will it cost?" Both of our primary sources for TBI injured individuals, the military and the gridiron, accrue these injuries as a part of their business-as-usual. My belief is that every one of us reading this needs to lift our voices and remind these organizations' leaders that, as Lipton mentioned, prevention is preferred. It would be much more cost-effective to admit to the problem, invest in research to solve the problem, or prevent it altogether, instead of investing in media propaganda and legal defenses.

Next on our list is to prove that a seamless transition from the military to the civilian world is possible and can be very productive, not just for the veterans, but for the nation's economy. With assistance from Cardinal Health and the University of Southern California, we will find a way to collaborate with our communities and stakeholders to make this happen. If we don't, everyone ultimately loses—not just the battle, but the war. We can't continue to put veterans and athletes suffering from TBI and all the related symptoms out on the streets, leaving it up to emergency services—the most expensive of services—to pick up the pieces.

In the near future, we must develop diagnostic testing and long term protocols to track the benefits of the brain therapy, as well as determine the potential progress of the brain injury as the patient ages. Currently, there is no blood or spinal fluid test, no biomarker, and no radiographic protocol to detect changes in the brain with age. It is not acceptable that a patient progresses from "mild" TBI to chronic traumatic encephalopathy, a diagnosis made at autopsy, without some form of follow up for the years following the incident. There are current investigations into what type of diagnostics may be most successful in defining the post injury course. Serial modified neuropsychological testing has been advocated by some researchers in southern Michigan,[73] as well as researchers in Australia.[74] Most disturbing is the attention deficit and slower reaction time which may progress as a result of further brain tissue deterioration. Other researchers, including neuroradiologist Michael Lipton, are advocating serial diffusion tensor imaging of the brain with prospective, long term studies to determine even subtle changes in brain diffusion.[75] Still other academic institutions are pursuing blood test biomarkers,[76,77] while several scientific studies are underway to develop markers in the cerebral spinal fluid (CSF) surrounding the brain obtainable by serial lumbar puncture procedures.[78] However, the broad scope of a brain injury, including differences in genetic predisposition, differences in age and sex, different exposures to external forces, and differences in early treatment and management, requires the type of cooperative efforts we are noting from our global researchers on this issue.

Needless to say, multicenter, academic, cohesive studies are ongoing and swiftly gaining recognition in importance and urgency. Longitudinal studies of patients' recovery courses over decades are needed and are, in fact, already ongoing through efforts such as that of David Brody,[79] and Ann McKee, MD, primarily in the military world and athletic world, though interaction with all patients is encouraged. The TBI epidemic and the subtle, long term consequences must be documented and understood before they can be prevented. Dr. Ann McKee summarized the current research findings leading to progression of chronic traumatic encephalopathy in her December 2012 article published in *Brain*.[80] This article describes the processes of brain deterioration noted in CTE versus Alzheimer's disease. Continued research may soon lead to a protocol whereby risk of increased injury is easier to assess. If we can recognize the mechanism causing progressive injury, then perhaps we can stop it or at least slow the process down.

Understanding the effects of military-related mTBI presents numerous challenges. Military mTBI is diverse and difficult to assess, and no validated, objective biomarkers of the acute injury exist. Acute mTBI, whether from a concussion or a blast, is characterized by physical changes in the brain, including multifocal axonal injury, microvascular damage, neuroinflammation, and elevations in the protein known as p-tau. McKee and Robinson noted that although these changes are "considered to be reversible and to improve or resolve with time and rest, no well-established methods to monitor status or judge prognosis have yet been identified." [81]

Dr. McKee's assessment speaks to the cooperative efforts required, and it appears that these are ongoing within both the private sector and the government health care systems. The Department of Veterans Affairs announced in early 2017 that 1100 veterans who sustained TBI in Iraq and Afghanistan are to be followed for over 20 years.

Dr. William Walker, a TBI expert at the Hunter Holmes McGuire Veterans Administration Medical Center and Virginia

Commonwealth University, is leading the new study. He says the long-term observational study is one of the most comprehensive TBI projects to date regarding size, scope, and rigor.

Veterans Affairs sites in Houston, Tampa, San Antonio, and Richmond are enrolling in the study, as well as a defense site, the National Center for the Intrepid at Fort Belvoir in Virginia. An additional three VA sites will begin enrolling in the spring in Boston, Minneapolis, and Portland. The VA-Defense study aims to track mild TBI over decades starting February 9, 2017.

I have always struggled with the "ask" in presentations and interactions, especially because I truly understand that many Americans assume that this epidemic health issue is being managed by our government resources. I realize that, in some way, I've written well over a hundred pages of ask. Yet, to close out this time, I want to challenge you to get involved. Get involved in becoming a proactive caregiver for your returning family member, friend, or church member, for that will require energy and skills to navigate the healthcare systems for TBI assistance. Get involved in researching legitimate charities and other resources in your community, and donate time and finances as available. Volunteer to talk to civic groups, employers, and families so that TBI awareness will eliminate current obstacles for diagnosis and treatment. Get involved and become a one-on-one, proactive advocate for the heroes suffering from TBI in your community. Get involved making or collecting donations, assisting researchers, and volunteering your time or other talents to deserving causes and campaigns. Honestly, to a TBI patient, your intervention, no matter how small a gesture in your eyes, may just be the saving grace in theirs. Be the light that they are searching for.

When I began this journey with our veterans, I recall viewing, for the first time, the words of Margaret Mead. These words were displayed on Santa Monica Beach, where I first filmed for the documentary. These words continue as a call for action every Sunday as displayed by the Veterans for Peace Organization who turn the beach into a memorial for our fallen heroes.

"Never doubt that a small group of thoughtful, committed citizens can change the world; indeed, it's the only thing that ever has."–Margaret Mead.

Be that light– Be that change– Be that healing force. That is my ask.

EPILOGUE

Story of the Taoist Sage

On his sixteenth birthday the sage's grandson captures a wild horse and brings it home with him. Seeing his return, the people in the village say to the sage, "Oh, how wonderful!"

The sage responds, "We'll see."

One day while trying to break the horse in and train it, the grandson is riding and gets thrown off the horse, breaking his leg. He's no longer able to walk, so upon hearing about it the villagers say to the sage, "How terrible!"

The sage responds, "We'll see."

Some time passes and the military men come to the village to recruit all young men for the war. All the other young men get sent off to fight, but the grandson can't fight because of his leg. The villagers say to the sage, "How wonderful!"

And yet again, the sage knowingly responds, "We'll see."

In the nearly two decades since quite literally hitting the wall, changing the course of my life forever, I've reflected on the sage and the contemplative question of "is this good, is this bad—we'll see." I still think of that day in awe because I'd survived many more significant assaults on my brain without the type of repercussions associated with this one accident. "Is this good, is this bad—we'll see." This recurrent thought makes me truly grateful I decided to dig in with what was left of my former self, and learn to embrace my new normal. In doing so I believe I've found that this *is good*. Anyone who knows about TBI understands that it is a slate of pluses and minuses—something is given and something is taken away—parts of the brain cease to function and other parts step up to the plate, so to speak, to get you through this game of life.

My life in TBI recovery is a constant source of irony for me, where I have learned that losing things I thought were so core to who I was have been replaced by new defining attributes. The polar opposite of what I expect to happen, what I expect to feel, and who I intended to be all becomes magnified in my attempt to recover and improve my damaged brain. The challenges continue to this day, though not on a moment-by-moment or day-by-day basis as in the beginning. I'm happy to report that overcoming challenges remains a significantly rewarding experience.

My nearly photographic memory is gone; even my ability to read and remember had disappeared for a while—it was truly devastating. In fact, right after the injury I could have dwelled much longer on my inability to even just read, I suppose; but I am an impatient spirit. While I have recounted the story of how I managed to recover my ability to read, more important was the opportunity this injury gave me to discover audio books. I now cherish my Audible reading room.

Professional reader Scott Brick, whose voice is as clear as any I've heard, with perfect cadence and crisp pronunciations, assists me even now with my speech pattern. Since my TBI my speech can become hesitant and choppy leaving me to feel a lack of confidence. Listening to Scott Brick, trying to mimic his cadence and clarity, has helped me become a better communicator. My initial loss of visual abilities gave me increased auditory abilities; my initial loss of speech altogether eventually molded me into a better communicator.

The passion for numbers continues to this day. I can no longer play number games, add columns of numbers in my head for sport, or add the grocery bill in my head at the register, but I remain fascinated by what I believe is the purest of the sciences—mathematics. *Is it good, is it bad* ... now I find myself dabbling with numerology instead and it brings me a similar joy. Numerology deals less with mathematics and more with the occult significance of numbers. I'm not a true believer in that aspect, but I am bewitched by the playful configuration of the potential significance of the symbolism displayed through the numbers I've always had such a love for. Replacing the science of math with the possibility of good fortune in a number sequence gives me a familiar pleasure. The irony is my enjoyment of the possibilities that numbers may influence my brain and my life, rather than my manipulation of numbers to impact outcomes.

As for my loss of mapping skills, well, my friends and relatives would confirm that I didn't have much sense of direction to begin with. Being unable to read a map was a great inconvenience as I began driving to events to speak about TBI for those still struggling for light. As I wrote earlier in this book, it wasn't until almost 11 years after my accident that the ability to use maps returned. Surprises like this make me joke that the brain clearly has a mind of its own!

Without a doubt, my greatest gift from this brain injury is the gift of the people I have met, and my intense resolve to use my reclaimed voice to share the stories of those who can't share it for themselves. Almost daily I'm reminded in news stories and other resources about how our military members, veterans, and their families have had their cries for help unanswered by the bureaucracy of our current health care system in the process of TBI diagnosis and treatment. There simply are not enough rehabilitation physicians with experience in TBI recovery to provide services for the nearly 750,000 veterans from Iraq and Afghanistan who struggle with some form of TBI or PTSD. I truly believe my purpose for recovery is to provide hope to those who still need to be properly diagnosed and treated.

I am not by nature extroverted at all. At first, my TBI only exacerbated my desire to keep to myself. For me, it was seeing the plight of our returning service personnel, veterans and their families reflected in my own recovery that encouraged me to move out of my comfort zone and into the company of the DoD, the VA, and the Fortune 500 companies who are now trying to tackle this silent epidemic. As I tell my heroes struggling with TBI and PTSD, I can only sympathize about the method of injury, but I can empathize with them regarding the consequences and most importantly, I can show them a path to recovery if they're willing to go the distance. Miracles can be made to happen in both small and big ways. When I could not utter an intelligible sound for weeks I never would've imagined that speaking at Ft. Sam Houston, or Ft. Belvoir Intrepid Center, or Capitol Hill would be in my future. When I never attended meetings at the hospital that involved more than a handful of colleagues in my past, I could never have imagined that now I would be collaborating with veterans' organizations, and both VA and civilian health care leaders who are fighting for these brave men and women. The chaos within me as I was struggling to regain my brain has been rallied into a desire to tame the chaos within others who are still suffering, and to encourage them to strive for their new balance in life as well.

We are in a global TBI epidemic. I am one of the luckiest survivors I know, and I am bound by duty to share my energy and my experience with those still in the dark. I am not the person I was once, and is it good? Yes, it is good. I embrace the new me as I continue to learn more daily about how the brain functions through how *my* brain functions.

I sometimes look back on that day in my life; that darkest, hopeless, most oppressive day on earth when I tried to figure a way out. When I see the concern of a veteran's family who doesn't know what to do, or the face of a child who doesn't quite recognize their parent injured in combat, or the light come on in a suffering veteran's eyes, I realize why I hit the wall. I now realize I temporarily lost my brain so that I could regain my sense of humanity. I temporarily lost the science of medicine so that I could once again practice the art of being a physician. That has made all the difference.

MYTHS OF TBI

Throughout the book we've tackled these myths one-by-one and often looked at them through multiple lenses. I hope that these myths can be debunked and dispelled through spreading the truth about TBI and getting that word out to a wide audience; this is an issue that is increasing exponentially and affects nearly everyone—either as a patient, caregiver, or acquaintance.

MYTH 1—YOU NEED TO BE KNOCKED OUT TO HAVE A BRAIN INJURY.

FALSE - Studies have revealed that even mild, jarring injuries such as a soccer header or hitting your head on the car door frame can result in TBI. Often, there is a dazed feeling that lasts for only a few seconds, but you do not have to be knocked out to suffer a TBI. Of course, the more severe the injury, the greater the risk of blacking out. The longer you are unconscious, as a general rule, the more likely that the injury is severe.

MYTH 2 - IF YOU ARE DAZED OR ONLY MILDLY KNOCKED OUT, YOU CAN RETURN TO NORMAL ACTIVITIES IMMEDIATELY.

FALSE - Multiple studies have revealed the fact that resting the brain is imperative to healing. That includes limiting the stimuli from light, noise, or physical and mental activity. This is why high school athletes who suffer concussions may not return to school immediately due to the difficulties they can experience with studying, which also impairs brain recovery. This impairment is an even greater concern for soldiers engaged in battle.

MYTH 3—A SMALL CONCUSSION WITHOUT NOTICEABLE EFFECTS IS NOTHING TO WORRY ABOUT.

FALSE - Every head injury needs to be evaluated, treated, and followed up on based on diagnosis. Studies have proven that the number-one predictor for a head injury is having had a previous head injury, even a very mild one. We also know that the effects of repetitive injuries are more than additive. In fact, there is an entire syndrome called "second impact syndrome," whereby the second concussion, in rapid succession from the first (i.e. within hours, days, or weeks) can lead to a more severe injury or even death.

MYTH 4—EVERYONE WITH A BRAIN INJURY WHO FEARS OR AVOIDS CROWDS HAS PTSD.

FALSE—Avoidance of crowds, department stores, supermarkets, etc., as well as avoiding light or loud noise, is a trait of PTSD but it is also a hallmark trait of TBI. This results from the injured brain's inability to filter information and stimuli. If a TBI sufferer experiences high activity areas the result is stimulus overload for the brain, creating an adrenaline release, which may lead to panic attacks and further avoidance of these activities.

MYTH 5—I CAN SELF-MEDICATE AWAY THE EFFECTS OF MY TBI WITH ALCOHOL, DRUGS, ETC.

FALSE—Studies have shown between 70 and 90 percent of TBI patients develop addiction problems related to self-medication. Self-medication, especially with alcohol, but also with a variety of drugs, is a hallmark of TBI. The initial use may help to reduce the brain overload typically related to the injury but over the long term can lead to significant social, financial, and legal problems. A combination of brain injury and addiction is a leading cause of the suicide and homelessness epidemic currently facing our injured heroes.

MYTH 6—I JUST HAVE A HEADACHE FOLLOWING MY INJURY, NOTHING SERIOUS; ASPIRIN OR ACETAMINOPHEN WILL HELP.

FALSE - The persistent headache resulting from TBI occurs as a warning and is often related to vascular instability in the brain. Migraine-type headaches are common with TBI and should be treated differently than a normal headache, one which can be mitigated using aspirin or acetaminophen for the symptoms. Aspirin can increase bleeding as it acts as an anti-coagulant, and acetaminophen used in high dosages or used regularly over a long period of time can lead to liver problems. Both of these issues can be exacerbated by alcohol, which is the number-one self-medicating drug for TBI. Any pain treatment following a TBI should be prescribed by a physician, even if it ends up being over-the-counter medicine.

MYTH 7—I CAN'T CONCENTRATE OR REMEMBER THINGS AFTER MY INJURY LIKE I USED TO, I MUST BE GOING CRAZY OR BE OUT OF MY MIND.

FALSE - You may be out of your brain, but you are *NOT* "crazy" or "out of your mind." Difficulty remembering things and concentrating are functions of the brain that may be affected by TBI. Recent advances using diffusion tensor MRI can show us the areas of the brain that are injured or deficient. In the brain, even a small area of injury can affect a significant function, as with a lesion in the speech center, for instance. It is imperative that these injuries be diagnosed so that proper treatment can be prescribed.

MYTH 8—MY CT SCAN AND MRI WERE NORMAL, SO I MUST NOT HAVE AN INJURY.

FALSE - Current standard imaging techniques such as the MRI and CT scan do not have the capability to show the lesions or damage in a majority (greater than 95 percent) of TBI cases. If you are experiencing some symptoms of TBI and an MRI or CT scan were done that didn't detect an injury, you may still have suffered a TBI. Newer imaging techniques such as diffusion tensor MRI, SPECT, and PET scans can better determine the extent of injury in persons with TBI. Neuropsychological testing, similar to tests done with athletes, can also help to determine functional difficulties and therefore help to identify the location of the brain injury.

MYTH 9—I STILL FEEL OUT OF SORTS SIX MONTHS AFTER MY BRAIN INJURY SO I WON'T EVER GET BETTER.

FALSE - The brain may continue to recover for up to two years after the injury, possibly longer. Nerve injury healing processes require time and patience, and new research is proving that the brain can continue to repair itself for several years. Brain retraining through speech therapy, and mind strategies such as computer games or other applications, can assist with the brain healing process by prompting the brain to lay down new pathways to perform the functions lost with the original injury. Physical exercise and balance training can also improve function and healing. Please consult your physician about the electronic devices and exercise programs that are best for you.

MYTH 10—I CANNOT WAIT TO BE FULLY RECOVERED AND MY OLD SELF AGAIN.

FALSE - Even mild traumatic brain injury can lead to a shift in brain function and personality. Usually, the period of loss of consciousness or decreased consciousness is often followed by a period of heightened awareness or hyperactivity, especially if you have been injured during a time in which you were adrenaline- and cortisol-charged, such as on the battlefield or the playing field. This may last for many months, and you and your family must be patient until the brain arrives at its new "steady state."

You may approximate your old self but there will likely be some differences. You and your family should not get discouraged, but understand the process and accept these changes as they occur. Many navigators in Iraq and Afghanistan, for instance, lose their ability to read maps and follow directions after IED blasts. Finding support and acceptance for these changes is the best strategy for overcoming any related frustration and depression or anger. As with any form of disability, our brain and our strategies for carrying on will compensate in other ways for what was lost as long as we're willing to be open to these changes.

WHERE TO FIND THE LIGHT SWITCH

RESOURCES USED IN DIAGNOSING TBI

RANCHO LOS AMIGOS SCALE[82]

Levels of Cognitive Functioning

Level I - No Response: Total Assistance

- Complete absence of observable change in behavior when presented visual, auditory, tactile, proprioceptive, vestibular or painful stimuli

Level II - Generalized Response: Total Assistance

- Demonstrates generalized reflex response to painful stimuli
- Responds to repeated auditory stimuli with increased or decreased activity

- Responds to external stimuli with physiological changes generalized, gross body movement and/or not purposeful vocalization
- Responses noted above may be same regardless of type and location of stimulation
- Responses may be significantly delayed

Level III - Localized Response: Total Assistance
- Demonstrates withdrawal or vocalization to painful stimuli
- Turns toward or away from auditory stimuli
- Blinks when strong light crosses visual field
- Follows moving object passed within visual field
- Responds to discomfort by pulling tubes or restraints
- Responds inconsistently to simple commands
- Responses directly related to type of stimulus
- May respond to some persons (especially family and friends) but not to others.

Level IV - Confused/Agitated: Maximal Assistance
- Alert and in heightened state of activity
- Purposeful attempts to remove restraints or tubes or crawl out of bed
- May perform motor activities such as sitting, reaching and walking but without any apparent purpose or upon another's request
- Very brief and usually non-purposeful moments of sustained alternatives and divided attention
- Absent short-term memory

- May cry out or scream out of proportion to stimulus even after its removal
- May exhibit aggressive or flight behavior
- Mood may swing from euphoric to hostile with no apparent relationship to environmental events
- Unable to cooperate with treatment efforts
- Verbalizations are frequently incoherent and/or inappropriate to activity or environment

Level V - Confused, Inappropriate Non-Agitated: Maximal Assistance

- Alert, not agitated but may wander randomly or with a vague intention of going home
- May become agitated in response to external stimulation, and/or lack of environmental structure
- Not oriented to person, place or time
- Frequent brief periods, non-purposeful sustained attention
- Severely impaired recent memory, with confusion of past and present in reaction to ongoing activity
- Absent goal directed, problem solving, self-monitoring behavior
- Often demonstrates inappropriate use of objects without external direction
- May be able to perform previously learned tasks when structured and cues provided
- Unable to learn new information
- Able to respond appropriately to simple commands fairly consistently with external structures and cues

- Responses to simple commands without external structure are random and non-purposeful in relation to command
- Able to converse on a social, automatic level for brief periods of time when provided external structure and cues
- Verbalizations about present events become inappropriate and confabulatory when external structure and cues are not provided

Level VI - Confused, Appropriate: Moderate Assistance
- Inconsistently oriented to person, time and place
- Able to attend to highly familiar tasks in non-distracting environment for 30 minutes with moderate redirection
- Remote memory has more depth and detail than recent memory
- Vague recognition of some staff
- Able to use assistive memory aide with maximum assistance
- Emerging awareness of appropriate response to self, family and basic needs
- Moderate assist to problem solve barriers to task completion
- Supervised for old learning (e.g. self care)
- Shows carry over for relearned familiar tasks (e.g. self care)
- Maximum assistance for new learning with little or no carry over
- Unaware of impairments, disabilities and safety risks

- Consistently follows simple directions
- Verbal expressions are appropriate in highly familiar and structured situations

Level VII - Automatic, Appropriate: Minimal Assistance for Daily Living Skills

- Consistently oriented to person and place, within highly familiar environments. Moderate assistance for orientation to time
- Able to attend to highly familiar tasks in a non-distraction environment for at least 30 minutes with minimal assist to complete tasks
- Minimal supervision for new learning
- Demonstrates carry over of new learning
- Initiates and carries out steps to complete familiar personal and household routine but has shallow recall of what he/she has been doing
- Able to monitor accuracy and completeness of each step in routine personal and household ADLs and modify plan with minimal assistance
- Superficial awareness of his/her condition but unaware of specific impairments and disabilities and the limits they place on his/her ability to safely, accurately and completely carry out his/her household, community, work and leisure ADLs
- Minimal supervision for safety in routine home and community activities
- Unrealistic planning for the future

- Unable to think about consequences of a decision or action
- Overestimates abilities
- Unaware of others' needs and feelings
- Oppositional/uncooperative
- Unable to recognize inappropriate social interaction behavior

Level VIII - Purposeful, Appropriate: Stand-By Assistance
- Consistently oriented to person, place and time
- Independently attends to and completes familiar tasks for 1 hour in distracting environments
- Able to recall and integrate past and recent events
- Uses assistive memory devices to recall daily schedule, "to do" lists and record critical information for later use with stand-by assistance
- Initiates and carries out steps to complete familiar personal, household, community, work and leisure routines with stand-by assistance and can modify the plan when needed with minimal assistance
- Requires no assistance once new tasks/activities are learned
- Aware of and acknowledges impairments and disabilities when they interfere with task completion but requires stand-by assistance to take appropriate corrective action
- Thinks about consequences of a decision or action with minimal assistance
- Overestimates or underestimates abilities

- Acknowledges others' needs and feelings and responds appropriately with minimal assistance
- Depressed
- Irritable
- Low frustration tolerance/easily angered
- Argumentative
- Self-centered
- Uncharacteristically dependent/independent
- Able to recognize and acknowledge inappropriate social interaction behavior while it is occurring and takes corrective action with minimal assistance

Level IX - Purposeful, Appropriate: Stand-By Assistance on Request
- Independently shifts back and forth between tasks and completes them accurately for at least two consecutive hours
- Uses assistive memory devices to recall daily schedule, "to do" lists and record critical information for later use with assistance when requested
- Initiates and carries out steps to complete familiar personal, household, work and leisure tasks independently and unfamiliar personal, household, work and leisure tasks with assistance when requested
- Aware of and acknowledges impairments and disabilities when they interfere with task completion and takes appropriate corrective action but requires stand-by assist to anticipate a problem before it occurs and take action to avoid it

- Able to think about consequences of decisions or actions with assistance when requested
- Accurately estimates abilities but requires stand-by assistance to adjust to task demands
- Acknowledges others' needs and feelings and responds appropriately with stand-by assistance
- Depression may continue
- May be easily irritable
- May have low frustration tolerance
- Able to self-monitor appropriateness of social interaction with stand-by assistance

Level X - Purposeful, Appropriate: Modified Independent

- Able to handle multiple tasks simultaneously in all environments but may require periodic breaks
- Able to independently procure, create and maintain own assistive memory devices
- Independently initiates and carries out steps to complete familiar and unfamiliar personal, household, community, work and leisure tasks but may require more than usual amount of time and/or compensatory strategies to complete them
- Anticipates impact of impairments and disabilities on ability to complete daily living tasks and takes action to avoid problems before they occur but may require more than usual amount of time and/or compensatory strategies
- Able to independently think about consequences of decisions or actions but may require more than usual

amount of time and/or compensatory strategies to select the appropriate decision or action

- Accurately estimates abilities and independently adjusts to task demands
- Able to recognize the needs and feelings of others and automatically respond in appropriate manner
- Periodic periods of depression may occur
- Irritability and low frustration tolerance when sick, fatigued and/or under emotional stress
- Social interaction behavior is consistently appropriate

DEPARTMENT OF VETERANS AFFAIRS: DEFINITION OF TRAUMATIC BRAIN INJURY[83]

http://benefits.va.gov/PREDISCHARGE/DOCS/disexm58.pdf

A traumatically induced structural injury and/or physiological disruption of brain function as a result of an external force that is indicated by new onset or worsening of at least one of the following clinical signs, immediately following the event:

- Any period of loss of or a decreased level of consciousness;
- Any loss of memory for events immediately before or after the injury;
- Any alteration in mental state at the time of the injury (confusion, disorientation, slowed thinking, etc.);
- Neurological deficits (weakness, loss of balance, change in vision, praxis, paresis/plegia, sensory loss, aphasia, etc.) that may or may not be transient;
- Intracranial lesion.

External forces may include any of the following events: the head being struck by an object, the head striking an object, the brain undergoing an acceleration/deceleration movement without direct external trauma to the head, a foreign body penetrating the brain, forces generated from events such as a blast or explosion, or other force yet to be defined.

The above criteria define the event of a traumatic brain injury (TBI). Sequelae of TBI may resolve quickly, within minutes to hours after the neurological event, or they may persist longer. Some sequelae of TBI may be permanent. Most signs and symptoms will manifest immediately following the event. However, other signs and symptoms may be delayed from days to months (e.g., subdural hematoma, seizures, hydrocephalus, spasticity, etc.). Signs and symptoms may occur alone or in varying combinations and may result in a functional impairment. These signs and symptoms are not better explained by pre-existing conditions or other medical, neurological, or psychological causes except in cases of an exacerbation of a pre-existing condition. These generally fall into one or more of the three following categories:

- Physical: Headache, nausea, vomiting, dizziness, blurred vision, sleep disturbance, weakness, paresis/plegia, sensory loss, spasticity, aphasia, dysphagia, dysarthria, apraxia, balance disorders, disorders of coordination, seizure disorder.
- Cognitive: Attention, concentration, memory, speed of processing, new learning, planning, reasoning, judgment, executive control, self-awareness, language, abstract thinking.

- Behavioral/emotional: Depression, anxiety, agitation, irritability, impulsivity, aggression.

Note: The signs and symptoms listed above are typical of each category but are not an exhaustive list of all possible signs and symptoms.

SEVERITY OF BRAIN INJURY STRATIFICATION

Not all individuals exposed to an external force will sustain a TBI. TBI varies in severity, traditionally described as mild, moderate and severe. These categories are based on measures of length of unconsciousness, post-traumatic amnesia.

The trauma may cause structural damage or may produce more subtle damage that manifests by altered brain function, without structural damage that can be detected by traditional imaging studies such as Magnetic Resonance Imaging or Computed Tomography scanning. In addition to traditional imaging studies, other imaging techniques such as functional magnetic resonance imaging, diffusion tensor imaging, positron emission tomography scanning, as well as electrophysiological testing such as electroencephalography may be used to detect damage to or physiological alteration of brain function. In addition, altered brain function may be manifest by altered performance on neuropsychological or other standardized testing of function.

Acute injury severity is determined at the time of the injury, but this severity level, while having some prognostic value, does not necessarily reflect the patient's ultimate level of functioning.

It is recognized that serial assessments of the patient's cognitive, emotional, behavioral and social functioning are required.

- The patient is classified as mild/moderate/severe if he or she meets any of the criteria below within a particular severity level. If a patient meets criteria in more than one category of severity, the higher severity level is assigned.
- If it is not clinically possible to determine the brain injury level of severity because of medical complications (e.g., medically induced coma), other severity markers are required to make a determination of the severity of the brain injury.

MILD	MODERATE	SEVERE
Normal structural imaging	Normal or abnormal structural imaging	Normal or abnormal structural imaging
LOC = 0—30 min*	LOC > 30 min and < 24 hours	LOC > 24 hours
AOC = a moment up to 24 hours	AOC > 24 hours. Severity based on other criteria	
PTA = 0—1 day	PTA > 1 and < 7 days	PTA > 7 days

AOC—Alteration of consciousness/mental state / LOC—Loss of consciousness / PTA—Post-traumatic amnesia

It is recognized that the cognitive symptoms associated with post-traumatic stress disorder (PTSD) may overlap with symptoms of mild TBI. Differential diagnosis of brain injury and PTSD is required for accurate diagnosis and treatment.

SCHOOL OF PUBLIC HEALTH, UNIVERSITY AT ALBANY, STATE UNIVERSITY OF NEW YORK: PUBLIC HEALTH LIVE! IDENTIFYING AND ASSESSING MILD TRAUMATIC BRAIN INJURY: GUIDELINES FOR EMS AND HEALTH CARE PROVIDERS[84]

http://www.albany.edu/sph/cphce/phl_1215.shtml

"After watching this webcast participants will be able to:

- Describe the impact of brain injuries in New York State, including populations most affected
- Name at least three symptoms of mild TBI that can be determined through assessment steps in prehospital settings
- List the four steps of the pre-hospital assessment to determine the presence of a mild brain injury"

The University at Albany's School of Public Health offers educational programs through their "Public Health Live!" webcast series.

UPMC: UNIVERSITY OF PITTSBURGH MEDICAL CENTER SPORTS MEDICINE CONCUSSION PROGRAM

http://www.upmc.com/Services/sports-medicine/services/concussion/Pages/default.aspx

"The first of its kind when it opened its doors in 2000, the UPMC Sports Medicine Concussion Program is a global leader in testing, treating, and researching sports-related concussions.

"With over 17,000 patient visits each year, our more than 30 staff members treat high school, college, and pro athletes—including many from the MLB, NHL, and NFL—from across the United States."

In the Pittsburgh region, UPMC is a leader in health care; the Sports Medicine Concussion Program is a national leader in hands-on diagnosis and treatment in athletic injuries resulting in concussion. Additionally, some excellent information is available through their website.

RESOURCES FOR THOSE WITH TBI AND THEIR CAREGIVERS

THE OHIO STATE UNIVERSITY WEXNER MEDICAL CENTER/ OHIO VALLEY CENTER FOR BRAIN INJURY PREVENTION AND REHABILITATION: SUGGESTIONS FOR PROFESSIONALS WORKING WITH PERSONS WITH TBI[85]

1. Carefully observe and assess the person's unique communication and learning styles.
    a. Ask how well the person reads and writes; or evaluate via samples.
    b. Evaluate whether the individual is able to comprehend both written and spoken language.

c.   If someone is not able to speak (or speak easily), inquire as to alternate methods of expression (e.g., writing or gestures).

d.   Ask about and observe a person's attention span; be attuned to whether attention seems to change in busy versus quiet environments.

e.   Ask about and observe a person's capacity for new learning; inquire as to strengths and weaknesses or seek consultation to determine optimum approaches.

2.   Help the individual compensate for a changed learning style.

a.   Modify written material to make it concise and to the point.

b.   Paraphrase concepts, use concrete examples, incorporate visual aids, or otherwise present an idea in more than one way.

c.   If it helps, encourage the person to take notes or at least write down key points for later review and recall.

d.   Encourage the use of a calendar or planner. If the treatment program includes a daily schedule, make sure a "pocket version" is kept for easy reference.

e.   Write down homework assignments.

f.   After group sessions, meet individually to review main points.

g.   Provide assistance with homework or worksheets. Allow extra time for tasks that involve reading or writing.

h.   Ask family, friends, or other service providers to reinforce goals.

i.   Remember that something learned in one situation may not be generalized to another.

j.   Repeat, review, rehearse, repeat, review, rehearse.

3. Provide direct feedback regarding inappropriate behaviors.
   a. Let a person know a behavior is inappropriate. Do not assume the individual is making a conscious choice to act out or is even aware that he is misbehaving.
   b. Be clear about the behaviors that are expected and provide direct feedback when inappropriate behavior occurs.
   c. Redirect tangential or excessive speech, and establish a method to unobtrusively signal inappropriate behavior in public.

4. Remember that noncompliant behaviors may be symptoms of neurological deficits.
   d. Do not presume that non-compliance arises from lack of motivation or resistance. Check it out.
   e. Be aware that unawareness of deficits can arise as a result of specific damage to the brain and may not always be due to denial.
   f. Confrontation shuts down thinking and elicits rigidity; roll with resistance.
   g. Absences or lack of follow-through may be reasons to change treatment strategies. Don't rush to discharge.

UNITED STATES DEPARTMENT OF VETERANS AFFAIRS
https://www.va.gov/

The Veterans Affairs (VA) website is a portal to all services offered for returning US military members: information on health care and other benefits, locations of VA medical centers, and extensive information on research programs and support material.

RESURRECTING LIVES FOUNDATION

http://www.resurrectinglives.org/

> *"The mission: To coordinate and advocate for the successful transition to a post-military career and life for Veterans with Traumatic Brain Injury (TBI).*

> *"The vision: Veterans with Traumatic Brain Injury are properly diagnosed and supported during a successful transition to a post-military career and life."*

The Resurrecting Lives Foundation focuses on awareness, treatment, and employment for returning military members who have suffered TBIs. Tools and resources for the injured and their caregivers can be found through the RLF website, as well as a link to view the documentary "Operation Resurrection," cited in this book.

CONCUSSION LEGACY FOUNDATION

https://concussionfoundation.org/

> *"OUR MISSION: The Concussion Legacy Foundation (formerly the Sports Legacy Institute) is dedicated to advancing the study, treatment and prevention of the effects of brain trauma in athletes and other at-risk groups.*

> *"OUR VISION: Our vision is a world without CTE, and concussion safety without compromise.*

Focused on concussion in athletes, the Concussion Legacy Foundation has a rich website with links to educational materials, inspiring personal stories, links to local and national initiatives, and opportunities to participate.

STEPHEN A. COHEN MILITARY FAMILY CLINIC AT USC

https://militaryfamilyclinic.usc.edu/

> *"The Steven A. Cohen Military Family Clinic at USC provides individualized, holistic and timely mental health services to veterans and their families to improve quality of life.*
>
> *Through the national Cohen Veterans Network, our vision is to ensure that every veteran and family member is able to obtain access to high-quality, effective care that enables them to lead fulfilling and productive lives.*
>
> *"Who We Serve: All veterans (with a focus on post-9/11 veterans) and their family members. For us, a veteran is anyone who has served in the Armed Forces, regardless of role, discharge status or combat experience. This includes the National Guard and Reserves.*
>
> *"The clinic seeks to complement care provided by the Veterans Administration (VA) and to provide support for specific under-served groups:*
>
> - *Veterans who do not receive mental health care in the VA system*
> - *Veterans who have been denied care by the VA (e.g., due to discharge status, conditions that are not service-connected, etc.)*

- *Female veterans*
- *LGBTQ veterans and family members*
- *Veterans living in portions of Los Angeles County with few options for resources*
- *Veteran family members, including parents, spouses/partners, children, siblings and caretakers*

This groundbreaking clinic offers holistic support for military members and their families. While based in the Los Angeles, California area, they also sponsor a network of clinics across the country, accessible through their website.

UPMC - UNIVERSITY OF PITTSBURGH CENTER FOR MILITARY MEDICINE RESEARCH

http://www.cmmr.pitt.edu/

> *"Established in June 2012, The Center for Military Medicine Research (CMMR) 'represents a formal mechanism through which the challenges and opportunities of casualty care and wound healing can be examined at an advanced research level,' announced Arthur S. Levine, Pitt's senior vice chancellor for the health sciences and dean of the School of Medicine.*

> *"CMMR has lived up to Dr. Levine's pledge that the center would 'identify a network of successful partnerships and collaborations between scientists, clinicians, industry, and the U.S. Departments of Defense and Veterans Affairs to foster the most promising research technologies and therapeutic strategies.'"*

University of Pittsburgh Medical Center's CMMR is an example of the new collaborative research between government, industry, and science, driving research and education aimed at improving the care and treatment for returning injured service members.

CENTRE FOR NEURO SKILLS

http://neuroskills.com/

> *"Centre for Neuro Skills (CNS) provides medical treatment and rehabilitation, disease management, assisted and supported living, education, advocacy and research to achieve an optimal quality of life for people affected by brain injury.*
>
> *Our vision is to position Centre for Neuro Skills (CNS) as a world leader in medical treatment, rehabilitation, and disease management for individuals with brain injury, while pursuing and advancing the best clinical treatment, education, and research."*

With locations in California and Texas, CNS provides many treatment and support services, as well as online support resources through their website.

UNIVERSITY OF SOUTHERN CALIFORNIA SUZANNE DWORAK-PECK SCHOOL OF SOCIAL WORK PROGRAM IN MILITARY SOCIAL WORK

https://msw.usc.edu/academic/electives-options/military-social-work/

"The Military Social Work program option is designed to complement any department and will prepare you to:

- *Care for service members, veterans and their families who are dealing with a range of physical, mental and psychosocial issues.*
- *Better understand military culture.*
- *Learn about the systems of care in place for military personnel before and during deployments and the transition back home.*
- *Assist returning service members with finding health and employment services.*
- *Work with local agencies to identify and serve military populations in their communities.*

"Social workers trained in the Military Social Work program option work in a range of settings, offering services such as:

- *Mental health therapy, from physical illness and disease to family issues and traumatic experiences*
- *Military to civilian life reintegration support*
- *Crisis intervention*
- *Individual and family counseling*
- *Resource navigation, such as financial, housing and benefit assistance*
- *Aging veteran support and advocacy"*

Those involved in caregiving and support of our military can consider a military social work career through this unique program.

HOMEBASE

http://homebase.org/

"*Since our founding in 2009, Home Base, a partnership of the Red Sox Foundation and Massachusetts General Hospital, has been breaking new ground, leading regional and national efforts with a multi-disciplinary team of experts working together to help Post-9/11 Service Members, Veterans and their Families heal from the Invisible Wounds of War: traumatic brain injury (TBI), post-traumatic stress (PTS), and related conditions. Today, Home Base is the only private sector clinic in New England, and the largest private sector clinic in America with the sole focus of helping at-risk Veterans and Military Families regain the lives they once had. By caring for Veterans in a family-based clinic, and by working in cooperation with the Veterans Administration (VA) and the Department of Defense (DoD), Home Base serves as a replicable model to promote the health and well-being of Veterans nationwide. Mass General serves as the medical leader for Home Base and is the top-ranked hospital nationwide as reported by U.S. News & World Report 2014-2015.*

"*Home Base services are specifically designed to overcome common barriers to care for returning Veterans. We provide care to all Veterans and Families, regardless of ability to pay or discharge status, and utilize a "three generation" model of care that extends to parents, children, and extended family members who are effectively integrated into care. Our integrated team of child and adult psychiatrists, clinical psychologists and neuropsychologists, nurses and nurse practitioners, physical medicine and rehabilitation*

specialists, licensed clinical social workers, addictions specialists,
and peer-to-peer outreach coordinators—all of whom are Veterans
and/or Family Members of the Post-9/11 wars—work together to
ensure that Veterans and their Families receive or are connected
to appropriate and uniquely-tailored care.

Based in Boston, Massachusetts, HomeBase offers care for military members and their families, and educational and support materials through their website.

...and all sources cited in this text

The extensive list of sources cited in this text (see Bibliography) include locations around the country; diagnosis, care options, and support services may be available nearby through consultation with these experts.

ONLINE SUPPORT FOR THOSE WITH TBI AND THEIR CAREGIVERS

BRAINLINE.ORG
http://www.brainline.org

> *"BrainLine is a national multimedia project offering information*
> *and resources about preventing, treating, and living with TBI.*
> *BrainLine includes a series of webcasts, an electronic newsletter,*
> *and an extensive outreach campaign in partnership with national*
> *organizations concerned about traumatic brain injury.*

"BrainLine serves anyone whose life has been affected by TBI. That includes people with brain injury, their families, professionals in the field, and anyone else in a position to help prevent or ameliorate the toll of TBI.

"Through BrainLine, we seek to provide a sense of community, a place where people who care about TBI can go 24 hours a day for information, support, and ideas."

BRAIN INJURY ASSOCIATION OF AMERICA

biaausa.org

"BIAA's mission is to advance awareness, research, treatment, and education and to improve the quality of life for all people affected by brain injury. We are dedicated to increasing access to quality health care and raising awareness and understanding of brain injury. With a network of state affiliates, local chapters, and support groups, we are the voice of brain injury."

Website links to many pages of online information, state-by-state contacts and websites, information on advocacy and government affairs, and links to resources for purchase

THE ELIZABETH DOLE FOUNDATION: CARING FOR MILITARY FAMILIES

http://www.elizabethdolefoundation.org/

"Thanks to advances in battlefield medicine, thousands of our troops who would have perished in past wars, are now surviving. However, many have devastating wounds, illnesses and injuries, both visible and invisible, requiring care long after they have left the military health care system. Who are their caregivers?

"They are spouses, parents, siblings and other loved ones performing a stunning array of functions at home. These caregivers are administering medications, navigating complex health care systems, providing emotional support, arranging rehabilitation, handling the family's legal and financial matters, and acting as advocates on behalf of those for whom they are caring. Many are also raising children and providing an income for the family.

"Military and veteran caregivers are an unpaid workforce saving our nation billions in health care costs and potential institutionalization. In some cases, the time demands of caretaking may result in lost jobs, lost wages, and possible loss of health insurance. Though caregiver needs are many, no national strategy for supporting them has existed. As they put the well being of their loved ones before their own, the physical and emotional toll on caregivers over months and years can be devastating."

Website is a clearinghouse of information in support of caregivers for military members.

NATIONAL RESOURCE CENTER FOR TRAUMATIC BRAIN INJURY

http://www.tbinrc.com/

"The mission of the National Resource Center for Traumatic Brain Injury (NRCTBI) is to provide relevant, practical information for professionals, persons with brain injury, and family members. We have more than two decades of experience investigating the special needs and problems of people with brain injury and their families. With input from consumers and nationally recognized experts, we have developed a wide variety of assessment tools, intervention programs, and training programs. The NRCTBI is housed at Virginia Commonwealth University's Medical College of Virginia Campus. Many of our staff are affiliated with the Virginia Commonwealth Traumatic Brain Injury Model System."

DEFENSE AND VETERANS BRAIN INJURY CENTER

http://dvbic.dcoe.mil/resources

"The Defense and Veterans Brain Injury Center (DVBIC) is a part of the U.S. Military Health System. Specifically, DVBIC is the traumatic brain injury (TBI) operational component of the Defense Centers of Excellence for Psychological Health and Traumatic Brain Injury (DCoE). Founded in 1992 by Congress, DVBIC's responsibilities have grown as its network of care and treatment sites has grown.

"DVBIC's mission is to serve active-duty military, their beneficiaries, and veterans with traumatic brain injury through state-of-the-science clinical care, innovative clinical research initiatives and

educational programs, and support for force health protection services. DVBIC fulfills this mission through ongoing collaboration with the Department of Defense (DoD), military services, Department of Veterans Affairs (VA), civilian health partners, local communities, families and individuals with TBI.

"At 18 sites supported by a Washington, D.C.-area headquarters, DVBIC treats, supports, trains and monitors service members, veterans, family members and providers who have been, or care for those who are, affected by traumatic brain injury.

"DVBIC works at the macro-level, screening and briefing troops heading into theater, performing pre-deployment provider training at military treatment facilities, gathering data mandated by Congress and DoD, and overseeing research programs. At the micro-level, DVBIC treats service members and veterans with mild, moderate or severe TBI, and helps them from the moment of injury to their return to duty or reintegration into the community. DVBIC develops, provides and distributes educational materials for both military and civilian providers, families, service members and veterans."

Website has a wealth of information, including links to research studies, support material for those suffering from TBI, and educational materials for professionals, caregivers, and family members.

THE TIRR FOUNDATION

http://www.tirrfoundation.org/

> *"The Institute for Rehabilitation and Research (TIRR) Foundation is a nonprofit 501 (c) 3 organization that seeks to improve the lives of people who have sustained central nervous system damage through injury or disease. TIRR Foundation created, directs and funds Mission Connect, a collaborative neurotrauma research project. Mission Connect is focused on supporting the discovery of preventions, treatments and cures for central nervous system damage caused by brain injuries, spinal cord injuries, and neurodegenerative diseases.*

> *"TIRR Foundation also supports youth programs including a summer camp and sports team for wheelchair dependent children and young adults. Furthermore, to aid with the rehabilitation of patients, TIRR Foundation provides funding to purchase critical equipment within one of Houston's premier rehabilitation outpatient clinics. In 2007, TIRR Foundation launched Project Victory, a brain injury research program that serves American military services members."*

TIRR and its research and support units offer programs for both military members and youth in the Houston, Texas area.

END NOTES

CHAPTER 1

1 Tanielian and Jaycox, *Invisible Wounds of War: Psychological and Cognitive Injuries, Their Consequences, and Services to Assist Recovery.*

2 Kirk, Gilmore, And Wiser, "League of Denial."

3 Taylor et al., "Traumatic Brain Injury—Related Emergency Department Visits, Hospitalizations, and Deaths—United States, 2007 and 2013."

4 Tanielian and Jaycox, *Invisible Wounds of War.*

5 Editor, Lancet Neurology, "The Changing Landscape of Traumatic Brain Injury Research."

6 Jaramillo, "More than 40% of Retired NFL Players Showed Evidence of Traumatic Brain Injury."

CHAPTER 2

7 Hagen, Malkmus, and Durham, "Levels of Cognitive Functioning."

8 Stippler et al., "Utility of Routine Follow-up Head CT Scanning after Mild Traumatic Brain Injury."

9 Gordon, *Operation Resurrection.*

CHAPTER 3

10 Keltner and Cooke, "Biological Perspectives Traumatic Brain Injury—War Related."

11 Baumann et al., "Loss of Hypocretin (Orexin) Neurons with Traumatic Brain Injury."

12 Scholz, DOCKET NO. 09-20 11 On appeal from the Department of Veterans Affairs Regional Office in San Diego, California THE ISSUE Entitlement to service connection for residuals of a traumatic brain injury (TBI).

13 Wylie et al., "Cognitive Improvement after Mild Traumatic Brain Injury Measured with Functional Neuroimaging during the Acute Period."

14 Topolovec-Vranic et al., "Traumatic Brain Injury among Men in an Urban Homeless Shelter."

15 National Coalition for Homeless Veterans, "National Coalition for Homeless Veterans - Background and Statistics."

16 Laich, *Skin in the Game.*

17 Mortimer, "French Study Looks at Frequency of Rugby Injuries by Position."

18 Branch, "Brandi Chastain to Donate Her Brain for C.T.E. Research."

19 Chappell, "U.S. Military's Suicide Rate Surpassed Combat Deaths in 2012."

20 Perez, "BMX Star Dave Mirra's Brain Showed Signs of CTE."

21 Laskas, *Concussion.*

22 Landesman, *Concussion.*

23 Joiner, *Why People Die by Suicide.*

24 BenGurion University and Joiner, *"Why Do People Die By Suicide" - Lecture by Thomas E. Joiner, Ph.D.*

25 Missouri Department of Health and Senior Services and Missouri University Department of Health Psychology, "Substance Use/Abuse and TBI | TBI Basics."

26 Breggin, *Exploring the Relationship Between Medication and Veteran Suicide.*

27 Breggin, "Chapter 10: TBI, PTSD, and Psychiatric Drugs: A Perfect Storm for Causing Abnormal Mental States and Aberrant Behavior."

28 Griffin, Charron, and Al-Daccak, "Post-Traumatic Stress Disorder."

CHAPTER 4

29 Brooks et al., "The Five Year Outcome of Severe Blunt Head Injury: A Relative's View."

30 Merritt Hawkins, "RVU Based Physician Compensation and Productivity."

31 Giacino et al., "Placebo-Controlled Trial of Amantadine for Severe Traumatic Brain Injury."

32 McKee et al., "The Spectrum of Disease in Chronic Traumatic Encephalopathy"; "Chronic Traumatic Encephalopathy."

33 Belson, "N.F.L. Official Affirms Link Between Playing Football and C.T.E."

34 Cardinale, "Traumatic Brain Injury: The Hidden Epidemic Nobody Wants to Talk About."

CHAPTER 5

35 Pomaville and Hilchey, "An 'Academic Prep Group' for Combat Veterans With TBI: Lessons Learned."

36 United States Department of Defense, "DoD Worldwide Numbers for TBI."

37 "CogSMART." http://www.cogsmart.com/

CHAPTER 6

38 Darabont, *The Shawshank Redemption.*

39 Albert Einstein College of Medicine and Lipton, *Science Talk*; Albert Einstein College

of Medicine and Lipton, "Novel Brain Imaging Technique Explains Why Concussions Affect People Differently."

40 "Always Get Home on the App Store."

41 Lange et al., "Development and Evaluation of Low Cost Game-Based Balance Rehabilitation Tool Using the Microsoft Kinect Sensor."

42 Freitas et al., "Development and Evaluation of a Kinect Based Motor Rehabilitation Game."

43 Wilson, "Video Games Show Promise as Therapy."

44 McGonigal, *The Game That Can Give You 10 Extra Years of Life.*

45 "SuperBetter." http://www.superbetter.com.

46 "MindMaze." http://www.mindmaze.com.

47 Golub and TBWA\Chiat\Day, *Apple Steve Jobs The Crazy Ones - NEVER BEFORE AIRED 1997 - (Original Post).*

CHAPTER 7

48 Gladwell, *Outliers.*

49 McClelland et al., "Detection of Blast-Related White Matter Injury in Iraq and Afghanistan Combat Veterans Is Modulated by Control Group Composition."

50 The Ohio State University Wexner Medical Center, Ohio Valley for Brain Injury Prevention and Rehabilitation, "Substance Use after TBI: Information for Consumers Ohio Valley Center for Brain Injury Prevention and Rehabilitation."

51 Bombardier and Turner, "Chapter 14: Alcohol and Other Drug Use in Traumatic Disability."

52 The Ohio State University Wexner Medical Center, Ohio Valley Center for Brain Injury Prevention and Rehabilitation, "Suggestions for Professionals Working with Persons with TBI."

CHAPTER 8

53 National Institute on Aging, National Institute of Health, "Neurons and Their Jobs."

54 Stufflebeam, "Neurons, Synapses, Action Potentials, and Neurotransmission - The Mind Project."

55 Dwortzan, "Professor and Paratrooper | BU Today | Boston University."

56 Woodruff and Woodruff, *In an Instant.*

57 Shively et al., "Characterisation of Interface Astroglial Scarring in the Human Brain after Blast Exposure."

58 "One Mind." http://onemind.org.

59 "LEADERS Interview with Peter W. Chiarelli, Chief Executive Officer, One Mind for Research."

60 Bey and Ostick, "Second Impact Syndrome."

61 Musser, "Time on the Brain."

CHAPTER 9

62 Saunders et al., "Pre-Existing Health Conditions and Repeat Traumatic Brain Injury."

63 Miller and Zwerdling, "Military Still Failing to Diagnose, Treat Brain Injuries."

64 Greenberg, "Veterans Psychological Health."

CHAPTER 10

65 Tanielian and Jaycox, *Invisible Wounds of War.*

66 Gordon, *Operation Resurrection.*

67 Belson, "N.F.L. Official Affirms Link Between Playing Football and C.T.E."

68 Hamilton, "How a Team of Elite Doctors Changed the Military's Stance on Brain Trauma."

69 Hamilton, "An Army Buddy's Call for Help Sends a Scientist on a Brain Injury Quest."

70 Parker et al., "Stretch-Induced Ventricular Arrhythmias During Acute Ischemia and Reperfusion."

71 Dwortzan, "Professor and Paratrooper | BU Today | Boston University."

CHAPTER 11

72 MacDonald et al., "Functional Status after Blast-Plus-Impact Complex Concussive Traumatic Brain Injury in Evacuated United States Military Personnel."

73 Podell et al., "Neuropsychological Assessment in Traumatic Brain Injury."

74 Collie et al., "Computerised Cognitive Assessment of Athletes with Sports Related Head Injury."

75 España et al., "Serial Assessment of Gray Matter Abnormalities After Sport-Related Concussion."

76 Meier et al., "Prospective Assessment of Acute Blood Markers of Brain Injury in Sport-Related Concussion."

77 Oliver et al., "A Season of American Football is not Associated with Changes in Plasma Tau."

78 Hicks et al., "Overlapping MicroRNA Expression in Saliva and Cerebrospinal Fluid Accurately Identifies Pediatric Traumatic Brain Injury."

79 Brody, "Mechanisms Underlying Tauopathy Following Traumatic Brain Injury."

80 McKee et al., "The Spectrum of Disease in Chronic Traumatic Encephalopathy."

81 McKee and Robinson, "Military-Related Traumatic Brain Injury and Neurodegeneration."

RESOURCES

82 Hagen, Malkmus, and Durham, "Levels of Cognitive Functioning."

83 United States Department of Veterans Affairs, "Traumatic Brain Injury (TBI) Examination: Comprehensive Version."

84 School of Public Health, University at Albany, Burns, and Kerr, "Identifying and Assessing Mild Traumatic Brain Injury: Guidelines for EMS and Health Care Providers."

85 The Ohio State University Wexner Medical Center, Ohio Valley Center for Brain Injury Prevention and Rehabilitation, "Suggestions for Professionals Working with Persons with TBI."

BIBLIOGRAPHY

Albert Einstein College of Medicine, and Michael Lipton. *Science Talk: Novel Brain Imaging Technique Explains Why Concussions Affect People Differently*. Science Talk. YouTube, 2012. https://www.youtube.com/watch?v=WEWA-PV90RM.

———. "Novel Brain Imaging Technique Explains Why Concussions Affect People Differently." *Albert Einstein College of Medicine*, June 8, 2012. http://www.einstein.yu.edu/news/releases/806/novel-brain-imaging-technique-explains-why-concussions-affect-people-differently/.

"Always Get Home on the App Store." *App Store*. https://itunes.apple.com/us/app/always-get-home/id1009613987?mt=8.

American Heart Association, American Stroke Association. "What You Should Know About Cerebral Aneurysms," November 14, 2016. http://www.strokeassociation.org/STROKEORG/AboutStroke/TypesofStroke/HemorrhagicBleeds/What-You-Should-Know-About-Cerebral-Aneurysms_UCM_310103_Article.jsp#.WMlEj_nyu00.

Baumann, Christian R., Claudio L. Bassetti, Philipp O. Valko, Johannes Haybaeck, Morten Keller, Erika Clark, Reto Stocker, Markus Tolnay, and Thomas E. Scammell. "Loss of Hypocretin (Orexin) Neurons with Traumatic Brain Injury." *Annals of Neurology* 66, no. 4 (October 2009): 555–59. doi:10.1002/ana.21836.

Belson, Ken. "N.F.L. Official Affirms Link Between Playing Football and C.T.E." *The New York Times*, March 14, 2016, Electronic edition. https://www.nytimes.com/2016/03/15/sports/football/nfl-official-affirms-link-with-cte.html.

BenGurionUniversity, and Thomas E. Joiner. *"Why Do People Die By Suicide" - Lecture by Thomas E. Joiner, Ph.D.* YouTube, 2016. https://www.youtube.com/watch?v=DESRIZtUIT4.

Bey, Tareg, and Brian Ostick. "Second Impact Syndrome." *Western Journal of Emergency Medicine* 10, no. 1 (February 2009): 6–10. http://www.ncbi.nlm.nih.gov/pmc/articles/PMC2672291/.

Bombardier, Charles H., and Aaron Turner. "Chapter 14: Alcohol and Other Drug Use in Traumatic Disability." In *Handbook of Rehabilitation Psychology, Edited by Robert G. Frank, Mitchell Rosenthal, and Bruce Caplan*, 2nd ed., 241–58. Washington, DC: American Psychological Association Press, 2010.

Borgaro, Susan R., Susan Gierok, Heather Caples, and Christina Kwasnica. "Fatigue After Brain Injury: Initial Reliability Study of the BNI Fatigue Scale." *Brain Injury* 18, no. 7 (July 2004): 685–90. doi:10.1080/02699050310001646080.

Branch, John. "Brandi Chastain to Donate Her Brain for C.T.E. Research." *The New York Times*, March 3, 2016, Electronic edition. https://www.nytimes.com/2016/03/04/sports/soccer/brandi-chastain-to-donate-her-brain-for-cte-research.html.

Breggin, Peter. "Chapter 10: TBI, PTSD, and Psychiatric Drugs: A Perfect Storm for Causing Abnormal Mental States and Aberrant Behavior." In *The Attorney's Guide to Defending Veterans in Criminal Court, Edited by Brockton D. Hunter and Ryan C. Else*, 714. Woburn, MA: Veterans Defense Project, 2014.

———. "Dr. Breggin Testifies Before Congressional Committee: Antidepressant-Induced Suicide, Violence and Mania: Implications for the Military." *Psychiatric Drug Facts with Peter R. Breggin MD*, February 24, 2010. http://breggin.com/dr-breggin-testifies-before-congressional-committee/.

———. *Exploring the Relationship Between Medication and Veteran Suicide*, Pub. L. No. Serial no. 111-62, § United States House of Representatives Committee on Veterans' Affairs (2010). https://veterans.house.gov/hearing-transcript/exploring-the-relationship-between-medication-and-veteran-suicide.

Brody, David L. "Mechanisms Underlying Tauopathy Following Traumatic Brain Injury." Research grant database. *Grantome*, 2017. http://grantome.com/grant/NIH/R01-NS065069-08.

Brooks, N, L Campsie, C Symington, A Beattie, and W McKinlay. "The Five Year Outcome of Severe Blunt Head Injury: A Relative's View." *Journal of Neurology, Neurosurgery & Psychiatry* 49, no. 7 (July 1, 1986): 764. doi:10.1136/jnnp.49.7.764.

Cardinale, Amanda Marie. "Traumatic Brain Injury: The Hidden Epidemic Nobody Wants to Talk About." *World of Psychology*, March 28, 2016. https://psychcentral.com/blog/archives/2016/03/28/traumatic-brain-injury-the-hidden-epidemic-nobody-wants-to-talk-about/.

Chappell, Bill. "U.S. Military's Suicide Rate Surpassed Combat Deaths in 2012." *The Two-Way: Breaking News from NPR*, January 14, 2013. http://www.npr.org/sections/thetwo-way/2013/01/14/169364733/u-s-militarys-suicide-rate-surpassed-combat-deaths-in-2012

"Chronic Traumatic Encephalopathy: Study Describes 68 CTE Cases in Veterans, High School, College and pro Athletes." ScienceDaily. https://www.sciencedaily.com/releases/2012/12/121203112808.htm

"CogSMART." http://www.cogsmart.com/

Collie, A, D Darby, and P Maruff. "Computerised Cognitive Assessment of Athletes with Sports Related Head Injury." *British Journal of Sports Medicine* 35, no. 5 (October 1, 2001): 297. doi:10.1136/bjsm.35.5.297.

Cooke, Brandi B., and Norman L. Keltner. "Biological Perspectives Traumatic Brain Injury—War Related: Part II." *Perspectives in Psychiatric Care* 44, no. 1 (January 1, 2008): 54–57. doi:10.1111/j.1744-6163.2008.00148.x.

Cronk, Terri Moon. "Military Leads in Treating Traumatic Brain Injury, Expert Says." *United States Department of Defense DoD News*, August 31, 2012. http:// archive.defense.gov/news/ newsarticle.aspx?id=117724.

Darabont, Frank. *The Shawshank Redemption*. [Film] 1994.

Dwortzan, Mark. "Professor and Paratrooper | BU Today | Boston University." *BU Today*, November 28, 2012. https://www.bu.edu/today/2012/professor-and-paratrooper/.

Editor, The Lancet Neurology. "The Changing Landscape of Traumatic Brain Injury Research." *The Lancet Neurology* 11, no. 8 (August 1, 2012): 651. doi:10.1016/ S1474-4422(12)70166-7.

Ehrmann, Max. "Desiderata." In *Wikipedia*, 1927. https://en.wikipedia.org/wiki/ Desiderata.

España, Lezlie Y., Ryan M. Lee, Josef M. Ling, Andreas Jeromin, Andrew R. Mayer, and Timothy B. Meier. "Serial Assessment of Gray Matter Abnormalities after Sport-Related Concussion." *Journal of Neurotrauma* 34, no. 22 (November 2017): 3143–52. doi:https://doi.org/10.1089/neu.2017.5002.

Freitas, Daniel Q., Alana E. F. Da Gama, Lucas Figueiredo, Thiago M. Chaves, Deborah Marques-Oliveira, Veronica Teichrieb, Cristiano Araujo, and Federal University of Pernambuco, Informatics Center, Voxar Labs; Federal University of Pernambuco, Physiotherapy Department, Applied Neuroscience Lab, Brazil. "Development and Evaluation of a Kinect Based Motor Rehabilitation Game." In *SBC-Proceedings of SBGames 2012*, 144–53, 2012.

Giacino, Joseph T., John Whyte, Emilia Bagiella, Kathleen Kalmar, Nancy Childs, Allen Khademi, Bernd Eifert, et al. "Placebo-Controlled Trial of Amantadine for Severe Traumatic Brain Injury." *New England Journal of Medicine* 366, no. 9 (March 1, 2012): 819–26. doi:10.1056/NEJMoa1102609.

Gladwell, Malcolm. *Outliers: The Story of Success*. 1st ed. New York: Little, Brown and Co, 2008.

Golub, Jennifer, and TBWA\Chiat\Day. *Apple Steve Jobs The Crazy Ones - NEVER BEFORE AIRED 1997 - (Original Post)*. Think Different. YouTube, 1997. https://www. youtube.com/watch?v=8rwsuXHA7RA.

Gordon, Chrisanne. *Operation Resurrection*. [Film], 2013.

Greenberg, Jeffrey. "Veterans Psychological Health: Spotlight on Our Service Members." *Altarum Institute*, October 9, 2012. http://altarum.org/health-policy-blog/ veterans-psychological-health-spotlight-on-our-service-members.

"Greg Louganis." In *Wikipedia*, N.d. https://en.wikipedia.org/w/index.php?title=Greg_Louganis&oldid=770314894.

Griffin, Gerald D, Dominique Charron, and Rheem Al-Daccak. "Post-Traumatic Stress Disorder: Revisiting Adrenergics, Glucocorticoids, Immune System Effects and Homeostasis." Clinical & Translational Immunology 3, no. 11 (November 14, 2014): e27. doi:10.1038/cti.2014.26.

Hagen, Chris, Danese Malkmus, and Patricia Durham. "Levels of Cognitive Functioning," in *Traumatic Brain Injury Resource Guide*. Rancho Los Amigos National Rehabilitation Center, Downey, California, rev. 1982, 1972.

Hamilton, Jon. "An Army Buddy's Call for Help Sends a Scientist on a Brain Injury Quest." *Morning Edition*. NPR, June 8, 2016. http://www.npr.org/sections/health-shots/2016/06/08/480608042/an-army-buddys-call-for-help-sends-a-scientist-on-brain-injury-quest.

———. "How a Team of Elite Doctors Changed the Military's Stance on Brain Trauma." *All Things Considered*. NPR, June 10, 2016. http://www.npr.org/sections/health-shots/2016/06/10/481568316/how-a-team-of-elite-doctors-changed-the-military-s-stance-on-brain-trauma.

Hicks, Steven D., Jeremiah Johnson, Molly C. Carney, Harry Bramley, Robert P. Olympia, Andrea C. Loeffert, and Neal J. Thomas. "Overlapping MicroRNA Expression in Saliva and Cerebrospinal Fluid Accurately Identifies Pediatric Traumatic Brain Injury." *Journal of Neurotrauma* 35, no. 1 (January 2018): 64–72. doi:10.1089/neu.2017.5111.

Jaramillo, Monica. "More Than 40% of Retired NFL Players Showed Evidence of Traumatic Brain Injury." *Healio Spine Surgery Today*, April 13, 2016. http://www.healio.com/spine-surgery/concussion/news/online/%7Bcbc2810d-ee17-4ccc-bce0-dce274d31893%7D/more-than-40-of-retired-nfl-players-showed-evidence-of-traumatic-brain-injury.

Joiner, Thomas E. *Why People Die by Suicide*. Cambridge, Massachusetts: Harvard University Press, 2007.

Keltner, Norman L., and Brandi B. Cooke. "Biological Perspectives Traumatic Brain Injury—War Related." *Perspectives in Psychiatric Care* 43, no. 4 (October 1, 2007): 223–26. doi:10.1111/j.1744-6163.2007.00138.x.

Kim, Namhee, Craig A. Branch, Mimi Kim, and Michael L. Lipton. "Whole Brain Approaches for Identification of Microstructural Abnormalities in Individual Patients: Comparison of Techniques Applied to Mild Traumatic Brain Injury." Edited by Pedro Antonio Valdes-Sosa. *PLoS ONE* 8, no. 3 (March 26, 2013): e59382.doi:10.1371/journal.pone.0059382.

Kime, Patricia. "American Legion Throws Weight Behind Marijuana Research." *Military Times*, September 8, 2016. http://www.militarytimes.com/articles/american-legion-presses-for-marijuana-rescheduling.

King, N. S., S. Crawford, F. J. Wenden, N. E. Moss, and D. T. Wade. "The Rivermead Post Concussion Symptoms Questionnaire: A Measure of Symptoms Commonly Experienced After Head Injury and Its Reliability." *Journal of Neurology* 242, no. 9 (September 1995): 587–92.

Kirk, Michael, Jim Gilmore, and Mike Wiser. "League of Denial: The NFL's Concussion Crisis." *Frontline*. PBS, October 8, 2013. http://www.pbs.org/wgbh/frontline/film/league-of-denial/.

Laich, Dennis. *Skin in the Game: Poor Kids and Patriots*. Bloomington, Indiana: iUniverse, 2013.

Landesman, Peter. *Concussion*. [Film], 2015.

Lange, Belinda, Chien-Yen Chang, Evan Suma, Bradley Newman, Albert Skip Rizzo, and Mark Bolas. "Development and Evaluation of Low Cost Game-Based Balance Rehabilitation Tool Using the Microsoft Kinect Sensor." *Conference Proceedings: ... Annual International Conference of the IEEE Engineering in Medicine and Biology Society. IEEE Engineering in Medicine and Biology Society. Annual Conference* 2011 (2011): 1831–34. doi:10.1109/IEMBS.2011.6090521.

Laskas, Jeanne Marie. *Concussion*. New York: Random House, 2015.

"LEADERS Interview with Peter W. Chiarelli, Chief Executive Officer, One Mind for Research." *Leaders Online*, June 2013. http://www.leadersmag.com/issues/2013.2_Apr/Making%20a%20Difference/LEADERS-Peter-Chiarelli-One-Mind-for-Research.html.

McClelland, Andrew C., Weiya Mu, Roman Fleysher, Namhee Kim, Mark Wagshul, Eva Cattenacio, and Michael L. Lipton. "Detection of Blast-Related White Matter Injury in Iraq and Afghanistan Combat Veterans Is Modulated by Control Group Composition." Montreal, Quebec, Canada: American Society of Neuroradiology 52nd Annual Meeting, 2014.

MacDonald, Christine L., Ann M. Johnson, Elliot C. Nelson, Nicole J. Werner, Raymond Fang, Stephen F. Flaherty, and David L. Brody. "Functional Status after Blast-Plus-Impact Complex Concussive Traumatic Brain Injury in Evacuated United States Military Personnel." *Journal of Neurotrauma* 31, no. 10 (May 15, 2014): 889–98. doi:10.1089/neu.2013.3173.

McGonigal, Jane. *The Game That Can Give You 10 Extra Years of Life*. TEDGlobal, 2012. https://www.ted.com/talks/jane_mcgonigal_the_game_that_can_give_you_10_extra_years_of_life.

McKee, Ann C., and Meghan E. Robinson. "Military-Related Traumatic Brain Injury and Neurodegeneration." *Alzheimer's & Dementia* 10, no. 3 (June 2014): S242–53. doi:10.1016/j.jalz.2014.04.003.

McKee, A. C., T. D. Stein, C. J. Nowinski, R. A. Stern, D. H. Daneshvar, V. E. Alvarez, H.-S. Lee, et al. "The Spectrum of Disease in Chronic Traumatic Encephalopathy." *Brain* 136, no. 1 (January 1, 2013): 43–64. doi:10.1093/brain/aws307.

Meier, Timothy B., Lindsay D. Nelson, Daniel L. Huber, Jeffrey J. Bazarian, Ronald L. Hayes, and Michael A. McCrea. "Prospective Assessment of Acute Blood Markers of Brain Injury in Sport-Related Concussion." *Journal of Neurotrauma* 34, no. 22 (November 15, 2017): 3134–42. doi:10.1089/neu.2017.5046.

Merritt Hawkins. "RVU Based Physician Compensation and Productivity." Merritt Hawkins, 2011. https://www.merritthawkins.com/pdf/mharvuword.pdf.

Miller, T. Christian, and Daniel Zwerdling. "Military Still Failing to Diagnose, Treat Brain Injuries." *All Things Considered*. NPR, June 8, 2010. http://www.npr. org/2010/06/08/127402993/military-still-failing-to-diagnose-treat-brain-injuries.

"MindMaze." https://www.mindmaze.com/.

Missouri Department of Health and Senior Services, and Missouri University Department of Health Psychology. "Substance Use/Abuse and TBI | TBI Basics." *The Brain Injury Guide & Resources*, 2012. http://braininjuryeducation. org/TBI-Basics/Substance-Abuse-and-TBI/.

Mortimer, Gavin. "French Study Looks at Frequency of Rugby Injuries by Position." *Rugby World*, February 16, 2016. http://www.rugbyworld.com/takingpart/ fitness-takingpart/study-in-france-reveals-findings-on-frequency-of-rugby-injuries-by-position-54325.

Musser, George. "Time on the Brain: How You Are Always Living In the Past, and Other Quirks of Perception." *Scientific American Blog Network*, September 15, 2011. https://blogs.scientificamerican.com/observations/time-on- the-brain-how-you-are-always-living-in-the-past-and-other-quirks-of-perception/.

National Coalition for Homeless Veterans. "Background and Statistics." *National Coalition for Homeless Veterans*. http://nchv.org/index.php/news/media/ background_and_statistics/.

National Institute on Aging, National Institute of Health. "Neurons and Their Jobs." National Institute of Health, 2008.

The Ohio State University Wexner Medical Center, Ohio Valley Center for Brain Injury Prevention and Rehabilitation. "Suggestions for Professionals Working with Persons with TBI." Columbus, Ohio : The Ohio State University Wexner Medical Center, Ohio Valley Center for Brain Injury Prevention and Rehabilitation, N.d.

———. "Substance Use after TBI: Information for Consumers Ohio Valley Center for Brain Injury Prevention and Rehabilitation," N.d. http://ohiovalley.org/ informationeducation/substanceuse/.

Oliver, Jonathan M., Margaret T. Jones, Anthony J. Anzalone, K. Michele Kirk, David A. Gable, Justin T. Repshas, Torie A. Johnson, Kina Höglund, Kaj Blennow, and Henrik Zetterberg. "A Season of American Football Is Not Associated with Changes in Plasma Tau." *Journal of Neurotrauma* 34, no. 23 (December 2017): 3295–3300. doi:10.1089/neu.2017.5064.

"One Mind." http://onemind.org.

Ontario Neurotrauma Foundation. "Guidelines for Concussion/mTBI & Persistent Symptoms: Second Edition | Ontario Neurotrauma Foundation." *Ontario Neurotrauma Foundation*, September 24, 2013. http://onf.org/documents/ guidelines-for-concussion-mtbi-persistent-symptoms-second-edition.

Parker, Kevin Kit, James A. Lavelle, L. Katherine Taylor, Zifa Wang, and David E. Hansen. "Stretch-Induced Ventricular Arrhythmias During Acute Ischemia and Reperfusion." *Journal of Applied Physiology (Bethesda, Md.: American Physiological Society)* 97, no. 1 (July 2004): 377–83. doi:10.1152/japplphysiol.01235.2001.

Perez, A.J. "BMX Star Dave Mirra's Brain Showed Signs of CTE." *USA Today*, May 24, 2016, Electronic edition, sec. Sports. http://www.usatoday.com/story/sports/actionsports/2016/05/24/bmx-star-dave-mirra-brain-injury-cte-suicide/84851622/.

Podell, Kenneth, Katherine Gifford, Dmitri Bougakov, and Elkhonon Goldberg. "Neuropsychological Assessment in Traumatic Brain Injury." *Traumatic Brain Injury: Defining Best Practice* 33, no. 4 (December 1, 2010): 855–76. doi:10.1016/j.psc.2010.08.003.

Pomaville, Fran, and Remy Sanchez Hilchey. "An 'Academic Prep Group' for Combat Veterans With TBI: Lessons Learned." Fresno State University, Communicative Disorders and Deaf Studies; Speech-Language Pathology Department, Veteran's Administration Hospital, Fresno, California, 2011.

Powell, Janet M., Joseph V. Ferraro, Sureyya S. Dikmen, Nancy R. Temkin, and Kathleen R. Bell. "Accuracy of Mild Traumatic Brain Injury Diagnosis." *Archives of Physical Medicine and Rehabilitation* 89, no. 8 (August 2008): 1550–55. doi:10.1016/j.apmr.2007.12.035.

Powell, Janet M., Elizabeth K. Wise, Jo Ann Brockway, Robert Fraser, Nancy Temkin, and Kathleen R. Bell. "Characteristics and Concerns of Caregivers of Adults With Traumatic Brain Injury." *The Journal of Head Trauma Rehabilitation* 32, no. 1 (February 2017): E33–41. doi:10.1097/HTR.0000000000000219.

Saunders, Lee L., Anbesaw W. Selassie, Elizabeth G. Hill, Michael D. Horner, Joyce S. Nicholas, Daniel T. Lackland, and John D. Corrigan. "Pre-Existing Health Conditions and Repeat Traumatic Brain Injury." *Archives of Physical Medicine and Rehabilitation* 90, no. 11 (November 2009): 1853–59. doi:10.1016/j.apmr.2009.05.020.

Scholz, Ronald W., Veterans Law Judge, Board of Veterans' Appeals. Citation Nr: 1107243 Decision Date: 02/23/11 DOCKET NO. 09-20 11 On appeal from the Department of Veterans Affairs Regional Office in San Diego, California THE ISSUE Entitlement to service connection for residuals of a traumatic brain injury (TBI)., No. 09–20 11 (Board of Veterans' Appeals February 23, 2011).

Shively, Sharon Baughman, Iren Horkayne-Szakaly, Robert V. Jones, James P. Kelly, Regina C. Armstrong, and Daniel P. Perl. "Characterisation of Interface Astroglial Scarring in the Human Brain After Blast Exposure: A Post-Mortem Case Series." *The Lancet Neurology* 15, no. 9 (August 1, 2016): 944–53. doi:10.1016/S1474- 4422(16)30057-6.

State University of New York, University at Albany, School of Public Health. Lee Burns and Hamish Kerr. "Identifying and Assessing Mild Traumatic Brain Injury: Guidelines for EMS and Health Care Providers." *Public Health Live!*, December 17, 2015. http://www.albany.edu/sph/cphce/phl_1215.shtml.

Stippler, Martina, Carl Smith, A. Robb McLean, Andrew Carlson, Sarah Morley, Cristina Murray-Krezan, Jessica Kraynik, and George Kennedy. "Utility of Routine Follow-up Head CT Scanning After Mild Traumatic Brain Injury: A Systematic Review of the Literature." *Emergency Medicine Journal: EMJ* 29, no. 7 (July 2012): 528–32. doi:10.1136/emermed-2011-200162.

"Study: More than 40 Percent of Retired NFL Players Had Brain Injury." *AAN.com*, April 11, 2016. https://www.aan.com/pressroom/home/pressrelease/1453.

Stufflebeam, Robert. "Neurons, Synapses, Action Potentials, and Neurotransmission - The Mind Project," 2008. http://www.mind.ilstu.edu/curriculum/neurons_intro/neurons_intro.php.

"SuperBetter." https://www.superbetter.com/.

Tanielian, Terri, and Lisa H. Jaycox, eds. *Invisible Wounds of War: Psychological and Cognitive Injuries, Their Consequences, and Services to Assist Recovery.* Santa Monica, California: RAND Corporation, 2008.

Taylor, Christopher A., Jeneita M. Bell, Matthew J. Breiding, and Likang Xu. "Traumatic Brain Injury—Related Emergency Department Visits, Hospitalizations, and Deaths — United States, 2007 and 2013." *MMWR. Surveillance Summaries* 66, no. SS-9 (March 17, 2017): 1–16. doi:10.15585/mmwr.ss6609a1.

Topolovec-Vranic, Jane, Naomi Ennis, Mackenzie Howatt, Donna Ouchterlony, Alicja Michalak, Cheryl Masanic, Angela Colantonio, et al. "Traumatic Brain Injury Among Men in an Urban Homeless Shelter: Observational Study of Rates and Mechanisms of Injury." *CMAJ Open* 2, no. 2 (April 1, 2014): E69–76. doi:10.9778/cmajo.20130046.

Twamley, Elizabeth W., Amy J. Jak, Dean C. Delis, Mark W. Bondi, and James B. Lohr. "Cognitive Symptom Management and Rehabilitation Therapy (CogSMART) for Veterans with Traumatic Brain Injury: Pilot Randomized Controlled Trial." *Journal of Rehabilitation Research and Development* 51, no. 1 (2014): 59– 70. doi:10.1682/JRRD.2013.01.0020.

United States Department of Veterans Affairs. "Secondary Service Connection for Diagnosable Illnesses Associated with Traumatic Brain Injury. Final Rule." *Federal Register* 78, no. 242 (December 17, 2013): 76196–209.

United States Department of Veterans Affairs. "Traumatic Brain Injury (TBI) Examination: Comprehensive Version." United States Department of Veterans Affairs, Veterans Benefits Administration, July 11, 2002.http://benefits.va.gov/PREDISCHARGE/DOCS/disexm58.pdf.

United States Department of Defense, Defense and Veterans Brain Injury Center. "DoD Worldwide Numbers for TBI." *Defense and Veterans Brain Injury Center (DVBIC)*, June 9, 2016. http://dvbic.dcoe.mil/dod-worldwide-numbers-tbi.

United States Department of Veterans Affairs, Office of Research and Development. "VA Research on Traumatic Brain Injury (TBI)." *United States Department of Veterans Affairs Office of Research and Development*, N.d. https://www.research.va.gov/topics/tbi.cfm.

Weinberger, Sharon. "Bombs' Hidden Impact: The Brain War." *Nature News* 477, no. 7365 (September 21, 2011): 390–93. doi:10.1038/477390a.

Wilson, Stephen. "Video Games Show Promise as Therapy." Text. *Military.com*, April 9, 2014. http://www.military.com/benefits/2014/04/09/video-games-show-promise-as-therapy.html.

Woodruff, Lee. *BUniverse: Life Changes in an Instant: A Caregiver's Journey.* Boston University: BUniverse, 2010. http://www.bu.edu/buniverse/view/?v=107tmbDT.

Woodruff, Lee, and Bob Woodruff. *In an Instant: A Family's Journey of Love and Healing.* 1st ed. New York: Random House, 2007.

Wylie, Glenn R., Kalev Freeman, Alex Thomas, Marina Shpaner, Michael OKeefe, Richard Watts, and Magdalena R. Naylor. "Cognitive Improvement after Mild Traumatic Brain Injury Measured with Functional Neuroimaging during the Acute Period." *PLoS ONE* 10, no. 5 (May 11, 2015): e0126110. doi:10.1371/journal.pone.0126110.

Zoroya, Gregg. "VA Suicide Hotline in Oscar-Winning Documentary Lets Calls Go to Voicemail." *USA Today*, February 15, 2016, Electronic edition. http://www.usatoday.com/story/news/nation/2016/02/15/va-suicide-hotline-oscar-winning-documentary-lets-calls-go-voicemail/80403618/.

Zwerdling, Daniel, and T. Christian Miller. "Pentagon Shifts Its Story About Departure of Leader of Brain Injury Center." *The Two-Way: Breaking News from NPR*, June 30, 2010. http://www.npr.org/sections/thetwo-way/2010/06/30/128220760/pentagon-shifts-its-story-about-departure-of-leader-of-brain-injury-center.

Made in the USA
Coppell, TX
07 September 2023

21338992R00128